THE BANGOUR STORY

THE BANGOUR STORY

A History of Bangour Village and General Hospitals

W F Hendrie and D A D Macleod

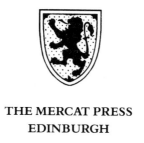

THE MERCAT PRESS
EDINBURGH

First published 1991 by Aberdeen University Press
Reprinted 1992 by Mercat Press
James Thin, 53 South Bridge, Edinburgh EH1 1YS

British Library Cataloguing in Publication Data

Hendrie, William F
    The Bangour story: a history of Bangour village
    and general hospitals.
    I. Title   II. Macleod, Donald A D
    362.1109411

    ISBN 1873644132

Typeset by BPCC-AUP Glasgow Ltd
Printed by Bookcraft (Bath) Limited

Foreword

Look to your health, and if you have it, praise God, and value it next to a good conscience; for health is the second blessing that we mortals are capable of; a blessing that money cannot buy.

Isaak Walton (1593–1683)

Thus wrote the author of *The Compleat Angler* and he must have enjoyed good health as he lived for 90 years.

One of his contemporaries was Sir Robert Sibbald, physician to Charles II and one of the Founder Fellows of the Royal College of Physicians of Edinburgh. He lived in West Lothian, the ruins of his home, Kipps Castle, are standing to the south of Cockleroy in the Bathgate Hills.

But West Lothian has a longer tradition than that of being involved in health care. The Knights of St John had their headquarters in Scotland at Torphichen where they had one of the earliest hospitals in Scotland. King David I of Scotland visited the Knights and the hospital at New Years Field in what was then Leving's Toun. The Knights recorded as important measures in the care of their patients, the availability of pure water, due attention to diet and the value of a herb garden. This herb garden was continued for several centuries and was later situated in Livingston on land near Howden. Sir Robert Sibbald recognising the value of this collection, was instrumental in bringing many of the plants to Edinburgh. These plants were originally in the garden at Nor' Loch, now Waverley Station and, subsequently, when this land was used for the railway station they were moved in the nineteenth century to what is now the Royal Botanical Gardens.

It was in the nineteenth century that a chemist in Linlithgow, David Waldie, first suggested chloroform for anaesthetics to Dr James Simpson, a famous gynaecologist who was born and brought up in Bathgate. Dr Simpson's achievements in helping to relieve pain during childbirth and operative procedures became internationally recognised.

Over the centuries there have been many contributions to the art of medicine from the area now called West Lothian, not least from those who have gone about the task of providing care and treatment for people when they become ill, quietly and unacclaimed.

v

Napoleon said that an army travels on its stomach. The names of the generals may be known, but the real heroes are those providing basic services. The same principle holds true in relation to health care, especially in the Bangour Hospitals.

Bangour was the estate upon which the Edinburgh Mental Asylum was established. The hospital was built utilising radical concepts of what we would now call a progressive care model and it provided treatment and care for 'the pauper lunatics' of the City of Edinburgh.

During two world wars it was the site for large military hospitals. After the Second World War the temporary buildings, which were part of the Emergency Medical Scheme plans for Britain, became the base for West Lothian's own general hospital services. This made it possible to provide a comprehensive clinical service with assessment, care and treatment available for psychological and physical illnesses and the associated distress. These hospitals have become, in the years since the inception of the National Health Service, very much a 'people's' hospital. They have continued to pioneer advances in health care, particularly in the integration of the different disciplines necessary for modern care provision.

Those of us fortunate enough to have lived and worked in West Lothian look forward to the continuation of services initially associated with Bangour and now based at St John's Hospital at Howden. But the most important point to appreciate is the real integration, over the past forty years, of primary care and specialist services. Primary care is the backbone of the Health Service. Without general practitioners, community-based nurses and related professions such as physiotherapists and occupational therapists, a comprehensive service could not exist. West Lothian, and the experiments in the provision of health care pioneered and developed in Livingston New Town, have shown how to integrate hospital-based services with the vital primary components. Inevitably, this book records the achievements in the development of psychiatry, surgery, medicine, obstetrics, the eradication of tuberculosis and many aspects of the complex care possible within a National Health Service. Perhaps at a later date the development of community services will be the subject of another book?

The authors of this history wish to express their profound gratitude for the countless stories, anecdotes, mounds of information and photographs made available to them.

We, the readers, must express thanks to Mr W F Hendrie and Mr D A D Macleod for their hard work, enthusiasm and drive which have made this book a source of so much fascinating information.

I hope you enjoy reading about your hospitals and your health service.

DR ALASDAIR A MCKECHNIE,
Vice-Chairman Mental Welfare Commission for Scotland
Formerly Physician Superintendent Bangour Village Hospital

Contents

List of Illustrations

Acknowledgements

We would like to acknowledge the tremendous help we have received from patients and hospital staff—both past and present—as well as the community in West Lothian, in writing *The Bangour Story*. We also thank the West Lothian Unit Administration for their support.

Individuals who have assisted us are too numerous to mention by name but many are identified within the text. We particularly acknowledge the help we received from Dr James Hendry, Physician Superintendent and Consultant Forensic Psychiatrist at Bangour Village Hospital, and Mr Colin Kirkwood of the Aberdeen University Press Ltd. On a note of sadness, we would additionally acknowledge the assistance of Dr George Summers who died recently, shortly after giving us a long interview about his years at Bangour.

Finally we would like to thank Rona Macleod, BA Hons Oxon, for her enthusiastic input in the closing stages, tying together all the loose ends and making last-minute corrections and Jane Swan for typing the manuscript.

As authors we have agreed that any funds or royalties that may accrue from the sale of this book will be paid into the Endowment Funds held in trust for the benefit of patients in the West Lothian Hospitals. We would hope, therefore, that you will enjoy this book and encourage its sales.

W F HENDRIE
D A D MACLEOD

Patrons

Publication of *The Bangour Story* would not have been possible without the very generous financial support we have received from a series of organisations and individuals. We believe that the generosity of this support is yet another manifestation of the high regard in which the Bangour Hospitals are held by the community they have served.

West Lothian Unit Endowment Funds
    Paul Taylor, Unit General Manager
Livingston Development Corporation
    James Pollock, Chief Executive
Surgicos Limited (a member of the Johnston & Johnston Group of Companies)
    W D Strachan, Managing Director
Ethicon Limited (a member of the Johnston & Johnston Group of Companies)
    G Borthwick, Managing Director
West Lothian District Council
    Councillor Dominic McAuley, Convenor
    Mr B Walker, Chief Librarian
Caesar & Howie, Solicitors, Bathgate
Sneddons SSC, Solicitors, Whitburn
The Scottish Society of the History of Medicine
    J S G Blair, President
Cameron Iron Works Ltd, Livingston
    J Beattie, Company Secretary
Kenneth Hogg LLB NP

Chapter One

The Hill of the Wild Goats

'Why do all this for the intellectually dead? How much better it would
be if we could do it for the intellectually living.'

With these controversial words the Right Honourable the Earl of Rosebery,
Lord Lieutenant of Linlithgowshire, officially opened the new Bangour
Village Hospital on 13 October 1906.

According to the reports of HM Commissioners in Lunacy, 'The Parish
of Edinburgh was erected into a Lunacy District on 29th January 1897.'
There was at the time great concern throughout the whole country at the
apparently rapid rise in the numbers of the mentally insane. While in previous
centuries every village had been reasonably happy to tolerate and accommodate its local idiot, the growth of cities during Victorian times con-
centrated the problem of the mentally ill and made it more noticeable and
much more difficult to deal with. By the end of Queen Victoria's long reign
in 1901, cities throughout Britain were being forced to face up to the problem
and, in the case of Edinburgh, it was decided that the creation of Bangour
Village Hospital was the answer.

Following the policy of the period, that the mentally insane could best be
provided for by isolating them in the country where they would benefit
from the peace, solitude and fresh air while at the same time being more
easily occupied labouring on the land, the Edinburgh District Lunacy Board
purchased in 1902 the 960 acre estate of Bangour. Situated 2 miles west of
Uphall and 4 miles east of Bathgate, Bangour was 14 miles from Edinburgh.
This was felt to be far enough away to satisfy the citizens' concerns about
safety but still within reach, especially by means of the private railway which
was planned from the outset, originally to carry building materials needed
for the construction of the new asylum but eventually to transport both
inmates and their visitors and the staff needed to care for them.

Bangour (literally translated from the ancient Celtic language as 'the hill
of the wild goats'), with its 200 acres of woodlands, set between 500 and 750
feet up on the south side of the Bathgate Hills, was originally the home of
the Scottish poet William Hamilton. Born in 1704 he was a descendant of

1

John Hamilton, who was a member of the War Committee for Linlithgow-shire in 1648. Hamilton began writing poetry while still a student and by the age of twenty he was a contributor to both the first and second parts of Allan Ramsay's *Tea Time Miscellany*, in which appeared, 'The Braes of Yarrow' and several of his other lyrical poems. During the 1740s Scotland was divided by the resurgence of support for the Jacobite cause and like all of his family before him, when Prince Charles Edward Stuart arrived in 1745 to try and relcaim the throne for his father, Hamilton took his side. After the Young Pretender's decisive defeat the following year at Culloden, Hamilton was forced to leave his home at Bangour and follow his Prince into exile. He remained abroad for three years, but in 1749 made his peace with the authorities and returned to his home in the Parish of Uphall. For the next few years Hamilton lived quietly at Bangour, but when he developed tuberculosis he decided, for the sake of his health, to return to France. The change of climate did not help and he died at Lyons in 1754 at the age of fifty. It is a strange coincidence that two centuries later Bangour became famous for its treatment of tuberculosis. Although today William Hamilton is largely forgotten, during the eighteenth and nineteenth centuries his lyrical verses were greatly admired and a complete edition of his works was pub-lished in 1850. His portrait, painted by Gavin Hamilton, hangs in the Scottish National Portrait Gallery in Queen Street, Edinburgh and the acclaim he enjoyed in his own time may be judged from the fact that Dr Johnson, while on his special journey to the Hebrides made an extra pilgrimage to visit Hamilton's birth place at Bangour. Furthermore, Hamilton's poem about Yarrow is said to have been the inspiration for the later works by Wordsworth, Hogg and Scott.

It is interesting to note that by the time Hamilton died in 1754 a new Bedlam House or Hospital had been opened in Edinburgh to house the city's insane. According to research undertaken by Dr A K M Macrae, the former well known Administrator of Bangour Village Hospital, the first provision which the city made for its mentally ill was as long ago as 1675 when several 'vaults' were constructed for them. These soon proved to be inadequate and three years later in 1678, an Act of Council provided for the construction of a 'Bedlam House or Hospitall' which was built in part of Greyfriars Yards, near where the statue of the famous Greyfriars Bobby now stands. It was under the control of the Governors of the Charity Workhouse and soon became very overcrowded, and was replaced in 1746 by a larger Bedlam which contained twenty-one cells accommodating sixty-four inmates, thirty of whom were described as 'pauper lunatics' and the other thirty-four as patients who paid £20 a year each for their upkeep.

During Edinburgh's Golden Age in the latter half of the eighteenth century many citizens became concerned about the conditions which even the new Bedlam offered and in 1792 a group of progressively minded townsfolk led by Dr Andrew Duncan issued a prospectus for a new Edinburgh Lunatic Asylum. It took over twenty years for their plans to reach fruition but in 1813 the new asylum was finally opened at Morningside. Patients or their relatives had to pay so this meant that the pauper lunatics lingered on in the old Bedlam at Greyfriars. Moves were made in 1819 to have them admitted to Morningside but it was not until 1844 that the managers of the asylum finally agreed to their admission.

Throughout the remainder of Victorian times the number of mentally insane in Edinburgh, as across the rest of the country, increased steadily, much to the concern of the general public who looked upon lunacy as a plague and worried about its spread very much as the spread of AIDS is feared today. Emergency wards were opened in the city's poor houses and batches of patients were boarded out at district asylums, but the super-intendents of these institutions protested about having to deal with 'Edin-burgh cases'. As a result, in 1897, by an order of the Secretary of State for Scotland, Edinburgh was constituted a Lunacy District and a District Lunacy Board was elected from the Edinburgh Parish Council. The Board appointed Sir John Sibbald as their Commissioner in Lunacy and Medical Adviser. He immediately advised them that he had no hesitation in recommending the construction of a segregated or village type of asylum. The members of the Board, however, decided that they must see for themselves and so set off on a tour of asylums not only in England but also in France and Germany. They were impressed particularly with the asylum of Alt-Scherbitz near Leipzig and decided that this was the place upon which Bangour should largely be modelled.

There followed several years of acrimonious planning with complaints of delay, incompetence, extravagance and about the management of the competition for architects. In the end Hippolyte J Blanc, RSA, was appointed, but he was warned, 'due to pressure on account of expense, to strip his elevations of practically all decorative ornament'.

The first buildings at Bangour were even more basic, because by 1902 the need for accommodation had become so acute and the Lunacy Com-missioners so pressing in their demands that the Edinburgh Board took action, and five temporary structures of iron and wood were hurriedly erected. On 1 June 1904 these were occupied by patients from the Royal Edinburgh Asylum. The first batch of patients consisted of twenty-seven women, but as soon as the second of the temporary buildings was ready they were followed by an intake of male patients. Other groups from both the Royal Edinburgh Asylum and several district asylums arrived during the next year and a half until by 31 December 1905, statistics show that all five of the temporary buildings were in use. Four of them were occupied to capacity by 200 patients—100 men and 100 women—while the fifth was par-titioned off to provide offices and sleeping accommodation for senior staff.

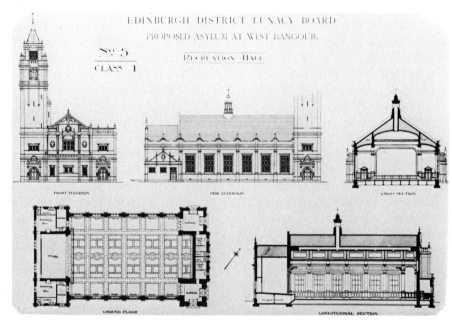

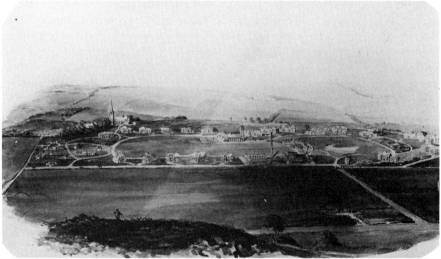

Figs: 1, 2 and (*facing page*) 3 How it all began. Plans, architects' drawings and a model prepared for the Edinburgh District Lunacy Board in 1902.

'Some estimate may be formed of the extent of the operations when it is noted that the length of the roads is 6,850 yards, or nearly 4 miles, and of drains, water mains, electricity cables, telephone wires etc, are together 28,180 yards—or over 16 miles.'

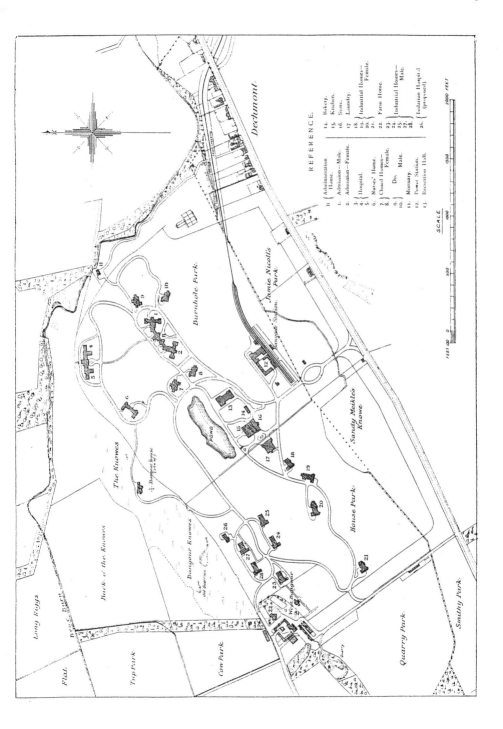

REFERENCE.

1. Administration House.
2. Admission—Male.
3. Admission—Female.
4. Hospital.
5. Hospital.
6. Nurses' Home.
7. Closed Homes—Female.
8. Do. Female.
9. Industrial Homes—Male.
10. Male.
11. Mortuary.
12. Power Station.
13. Recreation Hall.
14. Bakery.
15. Kitchen.
16. Store.
17. Laundry.
18. Industrial Homes—Female.
19. Female.
20. Female.
21. Female.
22. Farm Home.
23. Industrial Homes—Male.
24. Male.
25. Male.
27. Male.
28. Male.
26. Isolation Hospital (proposed).

SCALE

FEET 100 0   500   1000   1500   2000 FEET

Among the first residents was the newly appointed Medical Superintendent of the Asylum, an Ulsterman called John Keay who had until then been in charge of the asylum at Inverness. He provides a full description of the accommodation which he found waiting for him in his first annual report to the Board.

> The plans of these temporary villas, constructed by Messrs Wm. Bain and Co. of Coatbridge, were well thought out and their arrangements are convenient and workable. After residing in one of them for a year and a half, I can say that they are comfortable and healthy to live in. Owing to the nature of their construction however, they are easily damaged and it is feared that their upkeep in plaster and paint will be expensive.
>
> Since they were occupied, each of these five villas has had a verandah erected on the side facing south, at a cost of £475 for the five. These verandahs have been most useful. In summer the female patients practically lived in them during the day, the sewing machines being brought out and work being carried on in them as in a day room. To weakly patients also they are a great boon—those who cannot move about, even the bedridden—are carried out into the verandah, and get the benefit of the fresh air and sunshine.

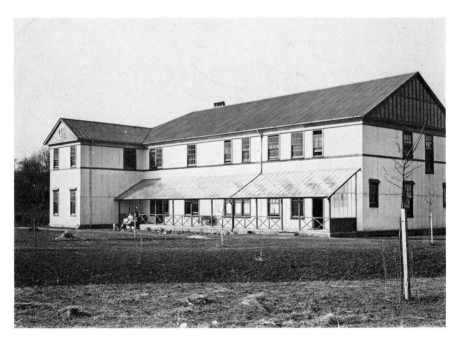

Fig. 4   Home 3, 1904. This was the first ward completed and opened for patients during the construction of the Village at Bangour.

Later in his report Dr Keay continues,

One of the homes for male patients containing fifty, and, among them, all of those confined to bed, or through illness or enfeeblement, requiring nursing, has been, since the opening, in charge of women nurses by night as well as by day. The employment of female nurses in certain male wards of asylums is now so usual and the advantages to the patients by the improved nursing so obvious, that it is unnecessary to do more than mention the fact that half of our male patients have been under the care of women since the place was opened.

In the organisation and equipment of the institution for the treatment and care of mental disease, no provision is of more importance than that of abundance of suitable occupations for the patients. In this matter, at least, Bangour will not be found wanting. On our large farm there will be found for practically any number of male patients for many years to come the most natural, health-giving and satisfying occupation available to man—cultivation of the land. Fifteen to twenty-six patients have been regularly employed at farm work, either as labourers on the fields or in tending cattle, pigs or horses. At busy times such as haymaking, harvest or potato lifting, the number is of course increased as required. Other patients have been employed in the garden, which is quickly coming into shape, or in the laying out of the grounds around the occupied villas. A nursery for young trees and shrubs, to be used in the future laying-out and planting of the grounds, has been formed and stocked, and a greenhouse for the supply of flowers and foliage plants to the wards has been built. To several kind friends we are indebted for presents of plants to fill this house.

Another feature of which Bangour was particularly proud was its private railway. Superintendent Keay reported:

The private railway, which had been in use for the carriage of building materials etc for a considerable time previously, was opened for passenger traffic on 19th June 1905 and has proved a great convenience to friends of patients and to the staff. The visiting day being Saturday, patients' friends get the advantage of the cheap fare given by the Railway Company on that day. It would be a boon to members of staff if they could have the privilege on any week day. Asylum workers are advised and encouraged for their health's sake to get away from their surroundings when off duty, and to mix with their friends in the outside world, but a young nurse, earning £18 a year, has to think twice before spending two shillings and five pence [12p] on her railway fare.

As an asylum Bangour was not unique in having its own private railway. Similar private lines were built at the County Mental Hospital Whittingham,

Lancashire, the East Sussex County Asylum at Hellingly and at the Stafford County Lunatic Asylum at Cheddleton. As in these English cases, the Bangour Railway was set up by a special Act of Parliament and as it was passed as early as 30 July 1900 it is obvious that the provision of the railway line was very much part of the original planning of the Village Hospital. Under the Act, the North British Railway Company agreed to operate the line, but the Edinburgh Lunacy Board was committed to a whole series of conditions, including laying the track, paying all overheads, promising to dismantle it if it ever ceased operation and guaranteeing 50 per cent of all revenue to a minimum of £1,500 to the railway company. The Act also laid down that from the point where the branch left the Edinburgh to Bathgate main line at a junction to the west of Uphall to the intermediate station at Dechmont the line was operated as a public railway, while from the village to Bangour it was regarded as private. The 1½ mile single track line was laid quite quickly and contractors' trains carrying building materials used it even before it was officially accepted by the old North British in 1903. A provisional time table was drawn up in 1904 but it was not until May 1905 that it was inspected by Lieutenant Colonel von Donop, Royal Engineers, and passed for general use with the first passenger train using it on 19 June. There was no special ceremony, but it was noted that the Bangour Station, which consisted of a timber clad building, was adorned with colourful hanging baskets cared for by the hospital gardener.

The 'Wee Bangour' or the 'Wee Bangour Express' as it was affectionately, if somewhat sarcastically, known—its top speed was 25 mph—usually consisted of three brick-red painted coaches hauled by a Drummond 4–4–0 tank No. 110 with solid leading wheels. There were three or four return journeys every day except Sundays with an extra run on Saturdays to cater for the many visitors. There was also one regular daily goods run carrying mainly coal and stores and, at Bangour, as well as the passenger platform there were three sidings which ran all the way to the low bank just before the main road entrance to the Hospital. One of the sidings allowed direct transfer of coal to the boiler house and to the east of the boiler house was a goods shed platform complete with a crane.

It was by the Bangour Railway that the guests arrived for the official opening of the Village Hospital on Wednesday, 3 October 1906. According to that week's *Courier*,

A special saloon train left the Waverley Station for Bangour at half past eleven and the large and representative company included Lord Provost Sir Robert Cranston and Lady Cranston, city officials and all the members of the Lunacy Board. On arrival at Bangour the company proceeded to the administrative block where the opening ceremony was performed by the noble Earl of Rosebery, who unlocked the door of the buildings with a gold key presented by the architect, Mr. Blanc. The company then walked through the admission wards, which are in this block and thereafter proceeded to the large store hall which was prettily decorated with flags and banners, where luncheon was served.

After the meal Lord Rosebery rose to propose a toast, 'Bangour Village' and said:

Bangour Asylum, or Bangour Village, as I think it is more happily called to remove the idea of an asylum, is one which I am told has been constructed on the most improved principles: that it is a model to all asylums of earlier date: and that it will be a resort of all those who are interested in such constructions. I have only seen a part of it, but I am quite sure that the airiness, the cleanliness, the cheerfulness and the spaciousness of the premises that I have inspected, that all has been said in its laudation is not extreme. But I have been asked not to dwell on the details of Bangour Village, but to propose the toast of Bangour Village. I confess that that leads me into a train of thought far wider, far more spacious, far higher, if I may say so than the details on which I have been dwelling. If I were to propose the toast of almost any other enterprise in the world, I should pray in all I said that it might be filled, that it might be occupied, that its sphere of influence might be indefinitely increased. Yet when I think of and look at Bangour Village, my hope and wish would be exactly the reverse, that it might be more a deserted village than the hamlet in Goldsmith's beautiful poem. And yet gentlemen we can see but little prospect of such a consummation. If we could see these buildings deserted for the simple reason that there were none to fill them, then there would be no happier or prouder day in the history of the kingdom. But what are the facts? I have brought here only two sets of facts; in the last reports of the Commissioners of Lunacy for England and Wales, they give these comparative statistics familiar to those who are at all intimate with the subject, which it is well to recall on such an occasion as this. On 1st January 1859, the total number of certified insane in England and Wales was 36,782 and on 1st January of this year 1906, 47 years afterwards, it was 121,979, practically 122,000. The rate in increase was equal to 231 per cent. You will observe that the figures exclude Scotland but I rather think that the figures from Scotland would offer an even more remarkable contrast. The general population during the same interval has increased at the rate of 75 per cent. Of course you must take from that deductions as to the greater willingness of people to put their relatives into asylums, and the greater stringency enforced as to insane people being kept at home, but nevertheless we have to face in these facts a certain and remarkable increase in lunacy; an increase which we have to face, the origin and source of which we do not seem entirely able to explore.

What an anxiety this lunacy is. What an expenditure on buildings and of money it represents. On January 1st 1904 the capital invested in lunatic asylums in the United Kingdom amounted to no less than £24m. The annual expenditure on the keeping of lunatics is £3½m and this is the huge barren fact that you have to face—this money is paid by the nation not for those from whom in the future it can have any hope or generally speaking in whom it can have any confidence as good citizens and subjects, but for those who represent sheer waste and decay. It is for this that we are building up these sepulchres of living humanity, these tombs of the intellectually dead.

Why do all this for the intellectually dead: how much better it would be if we could do it for the intellectually living? You are making sumptuous homes for the insane. Why, how many of the artisan classes would gladly change places with these lunatics? How few of the artisan classes can ever hope to have a home so sumptuous and so comfortable as these that you have made here? I believe the flower and blossom of municipal work will not have been reached until you have attempted at least to make a provision of living accommodation for the living and worthy workmen, for those who do deserve the comforts, which you have here extended to the intellectually ill. I am passing from the toast which I had originally to propose. I recall myself by a severe effort and I will ask you all to drink prosperity to the curative agencies of Bangour Village and the ultimate hope that the village may some day be found to be unnecessary.

Having spoken these prophetic words Lord Rosebery departed in his new-fangled motor car to be driven back to Dalmeny House, leaving a somewhat stunned audience to return to Edinburgh by train. Not surprisingly, next morning his Lordship's controversial remarks were headline news in newspapers throughout the country. Dr Keay had to wait until he made his annual report to the Board to reply to his Lordship, but this he did forcibly, claiming that the proportion of the population suffering from insanity had not grown, but was simply more noticeable because of changes ranging from the growing availability of suitable places to treat them, such as Bangour, to the terminology used in the 1901 census. 'People', he pointed out, 'who had an uncertified insane relative living at home with them did not mind entering him in the schedule as "feeble-minded", but they drew the line at calling him an "idiot",' which had been the expression used in all earlier census returned. Dr Keay also pointed out that better treatment meant that fewer mental patients were dying while the fact that many could be treated also ironically meant that fewer were being discharged, this again increasing the numbers.

Dr Keay's report also provides a full picture of permanent buildings at Bangour which were either ready for the official opening or were nearing completion:

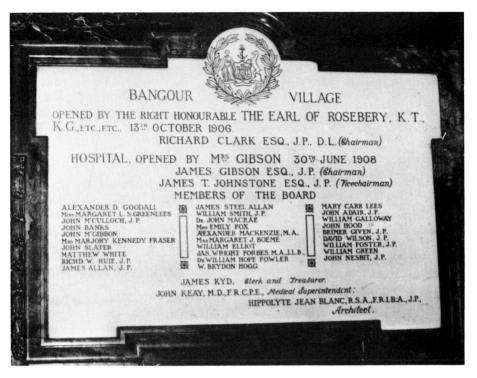

Fig. 5   The opening ceremony was commemorated with a striking plaque which
can still be seen in the administration block of the Village Hospital.

The year 1906 has been an eventful one in the history of the Institution
[he recorded]. A year's experience of the new Admission Wards and
the new Administration House has led one to form the opinion that
they are good buildings, having been suitably equipped and furnished
and will continue to serve efficiently the purposes for which they were
designed. The Admission Wards are in the meantime being used as
wards for the sick as well as for the newly admitted cases and will
continue to be so used until the hospital is ready for occupation which
will probably be about the close of 1907.

Dr Keay also noted all of Bangour's excellent facilities from the store's
newfangled cold storage chamber to the new bakery.

On the 2nd of July the new bakery was used for the first time and
since that date all the bread required in the Institution has been baked
in it, a very good loaf being produced at the cost of a little under a
penny a pound. The bakery has two ovens—one a draw oven of the

most modern description and the other a 'Scotch' oven of the kind that has been in general use in bakeries for a long period. The draw oven is the favorite with our bakers and is found most useful and convenient. The bakery is used for more than bread making. On one day of the week meat and potato pies are cooked there, on another day pork and on Fridays the fish dinner.

The central kitchen was opened on 8th September under the charge of Miss Archibald, who received her training at the Edinburgh School of Cookery and Domestic Economy. The kitchen is bright, roomy and well ventilated and the cooking appliances, which were supplied by the Carron Company are working satisfactorily. The food for the occupants of all the various buildings is cooked here, placed in suitable vessels and carried round in the specially designed wagon. Owing to the careful way in which the work of the kitchen staff is done, there has not been the slightest hitch, the food is invariably well cooked and reaches its destination hot and in excellent condition.

On Saturday 14th July the permanent laundry was occupied and the temporary structure near the wood and iron villas vacated. The laundry, with the adjacent home in which the patients and staff reside, is under the charge of Miss Grieve, who has been specially trained in this work. The machinery and appliances which have been installed in the laundry are believed to be the best of their kind, but irritating delays have occurred in the contractor's work, and at the end of the year it is not quite finished. Notwithstanding the almost constant presence of workmen, however, the work of the patients and staff has not been interrupted and has gone on smoothly from week to week.

The power station has been in full working order since 20th March and is under the charge of the engineer, Mr John Davidson, who keeps the plant in excellent condition. Steam is produced which is used in the laundry, kitchen and bakery to which buildings it is carried in a tunnel and electricity is generated for light and power wherever required all over the Institution.

(It is interesting to note that Mr Alistair Batchelor and other surgeons and their families living in the cottages in Dechmont still did not have electricity in 1950 and that their wives had to cope with lighting their homes with gas, Mrs Batchelor pleading with the Clerk of Works at the hospital to at least install special switches so that she did not have to keep the mantles lit all evening from the time it became dark!)

As well as envying Bangour Village its early supply of electricity, modern users may also envy the price at which it was produced for each unit cost only three half pennies, predecimal currency.

Returning to Dr Keay's report for 1906, the next buildings to be completed were the four 'industrial' homes for women, Nos. 18, 19, 20 and 21 on 8 November.

No. 18 is the residence for patients and staff employed in the laundry. The other three are occupied by patients employed at needlework etc. These four homes accommodate 190 patients and their nurses and are designed for the use of patients who are capable of being industrially employed. They are substantial stone buildings of pleasant appearance and yet absolutely plain and devoid of architectural embellishments. Internally in the finishing and decoration of the various rooms, the utmost regard has been paid to economy, while a bright and cheerful effect has been produced by staining and varnishing the woodwork and treating the plasterwalls and distemper in various shades. The furnishings are, as they ought to be, excellent, in design, in quality of material and in workmanship, without being in any sense luxurious or extravagant. A feature of these Industrial Homes is the absence as far as this can be attained, of arrangements suggestive of an asylum. There is not in any of them a bolt or bar or shuttered window. The doors open with ordinary handles. There is no padded room or single room in which a patient can be secluded from her fellows and liberty and freedom of action are allowed to the utmost extent consistent with safety.

Although Dr Keay does not mention it, Bangour always eschewed the use of any form of physical restraint and the straight jacket still used in many American asylums has always been regarded as strictly a museum exhibit at the Village Hospital.

For patients requiring special care and supervision Bangour had four closed villas. These were completed during 1907 and were designed with window restraints and other fitments so that those treated in them could not accidentally injure themselves. The secure units did not in any way detract from the openness of Bangour, a visitor at the time writing, 'no boundary walls enclose any of the houses nor are there any fenced areas, all roads and walks being open as in an ordinary village and the appearance is of an ordinary city suburb.'

This feel of a true village grew over the years with the addition of many features of a typical small community. The first of these was the erection in 1907 of a very fine Recreation Hall, complete with an excellent stage, orchestra pit and dance floor. The severe winter with its long periods of snow and frost which delayed the completion of the beautiful stone work of the Recreation Hall also delayed completion of the hospital and of the Nurses Home, the substantial four storey building conveniently situated close to the hospital block, the admission wards and the closed villas.

Another feature of the Village Hospital which always drew great praise was the farm. For instance, in his first report Dr Keay stated:

Although it has not as yet shown a favourable balance in the yearly accounts, the farm is amply fulfilling the first and most important function of an asylum farm, that is to provide healthy and congenial occupation for the patients. There is nothing that I know of in the treatment of the insane of more value and importance than occupation out of doors and there is absolutely no other occupation so natural, so soothing to the troubled mind and so health giving as that of farm labour. The profit on the working of the farm will come in time but in the meantime it should not be forgotten that, looked upon simply as a means of treatment, as a source of health to the jaded town workers who come to us, the farm is worth every penny that has been spent upon it.

The village has been supplied by the farm and garden with milk, beef, mutton, pork, bacon, oatmeal, potatoes and other vegetables. Extensive additions and alterations at the steading are in progress, having for their object the adaptation of this department to the future needs of the Institution. An airy and well proportioned byre has been built to accommodate 64 cows with conveniently situated apartments for the storing, and preparation of food, for the care of the vessels used in handling the milk and for the milk itself. A piggery for breeding stock is being built and the old byre of the farm is being converted into a house in which the pigs are to be fattened. It should be pointed out however that there is no implement house and on a farm conducted on modern lines the implements used are numerous and expensive. They soon deteriorate if they are not kept safely under cover when not in use. It is also recommended that a couple of sheds for hay and corn be erected in the stack yard. In this high district, harvest comes late and when it does it is of the utmost importance not to lose an hour in getting the crop under cover. A corn crop can be put into sheds in much less time than it takes to stack it outside; and not only that but it can be safely put into a shed when hardly ripe, whereas if built into stacks in that condition it would heat. With the use of sheds, of course, the labour and expense of thatching the stacks would be saved.

In his usual, persuasive way, Dr Keay, who seemed as good a farmer as a physician, got what he wanted. From these first early reports he was very much in control of the whole of Bangour Village and another feature in which he took a great pride was its pure water supply. This came from a reservoir constructed on the estate at the top of the hill, $1\frac{1}{2}$ miles above the village at an altitude of 700 feet, which gave a 200 foot head of pressure. The reservoir had a capacity of over 16,000,000 gallons of water and was calculated to provide 1,500 patients and staff with a supply of 70 gallons of water each day for five months. Later, during the First World War, it was to prove capable of supplying over 3,500 patients and staff even during the season of drought which left surrounding districts of West Lothian with a water shortage. The water was soft in character and so pure that it only required

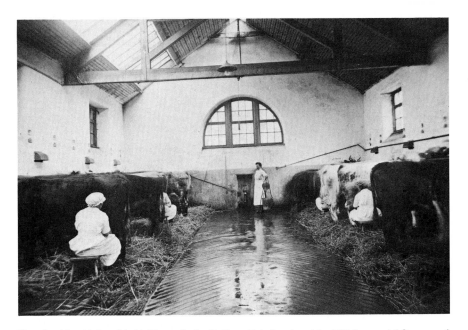

Fig. 6   Mrs Helen McNeillage (*née* Cathcart) left school in 1915, aged 18 years. A year later she came to work on the Bangour Home Farm at the Edinburgh War Hospital where her father, Col Charles Cathcart, was a surgeon working with the casualties from France. At the same time he developed his interests in spagnum moss for dressings, and the design of gas masks.

During her three happy years at Bangour, Helen Cathcart lived in the farm cottages. She was mainly involved in the byre, getting up each morning at 5.30 a.m. to milk cows and feed stock, including 300 pigs who thrived on scraps collected daily by a donkey cart from all the hospital wards. It was a long working day, helped by two or three other girls, half a dozen patients and some of the soldiers, with a cattleman and a farm manager in charge.

After her war service, Miss Cathcart went to college and graduated with a National Diploma in Dairying—with honours.

to pass through a series of sand filters before being drunk in the hospital. Keeping the water pure was also given as the reason for keeping the Bangour reservoir well stocked with trout, while of course this also provided a pleasant sport for the resident doctors on a summer evening. An attractively designed boat house was later added to complete this pleasant scene.

The reservoir was cared for by the waterman who lived with his family in a nearby cottage. His daughter Miss Allan still lives in Ecclesmachan and recalls her long walk to school in Uphall.

We were always getting into trouble for taking a short cut by walking along the railway line. When it snowed my father used to come down to help me through the drifts, but I was never short of companions for the Bangour Estate game-keeper also had a young daughter and there were always plenty of children at the farm cottages. We often met patients as we walked home through the grounds, but we were never afraid of them and always respected them.

Each year the number of patients at the Village Hospital continued to increase until by 1913 it reached 836. According to Dr Keay's report:

The ages of those admitted varied from 14 to 82, the average being in the case of male patients 50 and in the case of females 31 years. The great bulk of the cases, 126 out of 212 admissions were people in the prime of life between 30 and 60 years but 13 were over 70 and no fewer than 31 were over 60 years of age. There seems to be an increasing tendency to hand over to public care those in whom weak mindedness appears with the general decrepitude of old age, in the knowledge that they will be kindly treated and well looked after.

A large proportion of the patients admitted suffered from the more serious and less hopeful forms of mental disorder and were in an enfeebled state of bodily health. This is the usual experience in the case of mental patients drawn from a large urban community and it is most evident in places where the milder and more curable cases are intercepted and treated in general hospitals or observation wards. Included in the admissions were 10 cases of congenital idiocy or imbecility, 8 cases of acquired epilepsy in which the fits were accompanied by dangerous mental symptoms, 29 of general paralysis, 39 delusional or hallucinatory insanity and 39 of dementia or feeble mindedness occurring in connection with gross brain disease or as a result of former attacks of acute insanity, or in association with the general decay of old age.

The biggest difference between the admissions listed above for 1913 and the admissions for 1904 and earlier years was that instead of accepting patients from other institutions Bangour was now making its own direct admissions.

All the time improvements were being made and in 1914 plans were put in hand to provide additional lavatories for all the wards and metal roller blinds for all the verandahs which would allow them to be used all year round. The verandahs were indeed used all year round, but in very different circumstances from those which Dr Keay and his staff could have imagined.

Chapter Two

The Edinburgh War Hospital

'Negotiations have been completed for the taking over of Bangour Village by the War Office for the purposes of a great military hospital.' Thus reported the *Courier* of 30 May 1915 and great indeed was to be Bangour's role during the remainder of the First World War. Its accommodation was rapidly increased from just over 800 patients to 1,350 and it became the largest military hospital in Scotland.

As soon as the War Office decided that it required a large hospital in Scotland it was apparent that Bangour with all of its, at that time, very modern facilities, was their ideal choice. The District Board of Control agreed without hesitation and immediately plans were drawn up for the evacuation of the existing mental patients. A letter was sent to every other District Board in Scotland.

> The Board fully recognise [it stated] that in many asylums there is little or no vacant accommodation, that the staffs of various asylums have been depleted by the war, and that there is universal difficulty in obtaining the services of medical officers and suitable attendants. At the same time they expect to receive ready co-operation and assistance of the managers and officials of all institutions for the insane in the present national emergency, and they confidently hope that patients who may have to be transferred will be received into other asylums at the rates of maintenance current in these asylums or at a uniform rate, which may be fixed with the approval of the Board. In the meantime and in the special circumstances the Board will be prepared to relax somewhat the requirements as to the recognised floor space per patient in asylums.

The requested co-operation was forthcoming and so began what was virtually a military operation in itself to transport all of Bangour's inmates to their new homes for the duration. This task was aided greatly by Bangour's unique private railway, the existence of which was also one of the main reasons for its choice as Edinburgh War Hospital in the first place. Describing the evacuation of the mental patients the *Courier* of 21 May 1915 stated:

In regard to the removals to several of the West of Scotland asylums, a hospital train was used, the train making a round of all the institutions, switching freely from one railway system to another and dropping its quota at each of the stations on the list. In the course of next week a special train carrying as many as 350 patients will leave for the North. This itinerary will embrace 8 or 9 asylums, and it will therefore be seen that delay on the part of one institution in the completion of its arrangements would delay this whole scheme unless duplicate journeys were to be made. The special train in question will deposit patients at Cupar for the Fife County Asylum, and then will proceed by Dundee, Montrose, Aberdeen, Banff, Elgin and Inverness, dropping so many patients at each of these centres en route.

The *Courier* continues:

For transporting of the inmates to their new homes the War Office is responsible. In the case of removals to the Royal Asylum at Morningside, the work was done by means of Red Cross wagons, the patients in this case being mainly invalids. In the journey to Rosslynlee, another form of transport, the motor bus has been utilised and in the journey to Lochgilphead the various means of modern transport may possibly be exhausted, should it be decided to convey these patients by steamer.

It may be stated that the majority of the patients who can understand the situation accept their forced removal with equanimity, and several of them regard with undisguised satisfaction the prospect of a change of scenery and a consequent relief from what has been their daily routine during the last 8 or 9 years. It is the opinion of medical men that the change will do none of the patients the least harm, on the other hand it may do them a great deal of good. It must also be acknowledged that the friends of the patients recognising the national importance of the scheme, have no less heartily acquiesced in the new arrangements. Not a single complaint has been expressed in all the multitudinous correspondence which the scheme has occasioned on the part of the officials of the asylum and on the part of the relatives of the inmates. The chief concern of the friends has been that the patients should not be removed further from Edinburgh than is absolutely necessary and to such considerations Dr Keay, the Medical Superintendent and his assistants have given every attention.

For John Keay, his hospital's new role of War Hospital, brought the new title of Officer Commanding and he was granted the rank of Lieutenant Colonel to go with it. To his staff the Royal Army Medical Corp appointed Captain A C McMaster as Senior Resident Surgeon and Lieutenant H C Gibson as Senior Resident Physician together with six Resident Surgeons, six Resident Physicians and a Resident Dental Surgeon. Dr Laura Davidson was appointed pathologist, while the X-ray department was placed under the supervision of Mr Thomas Rankine. The nursing staff under Matron, Miss Isobel Davidson, was quickly increased to two hundred consisting of fifty sisters and 150 nurses and probationers and they were later to be assisted by fifty volunteers. The asylum attendants were also retained as ward orderlies and having taken courses in ambulance work were soon deemed, 'quite as efficient as RAMC orderlies'. Being an army establishment it was also considered necessary to mount a guard and this was provided by a sergeant and twelve men from the 9th Provisional Battalion Highland Light Infantry and they were accommodated in a large wooden hut containing 'a living room, sleeping quarters, bath room and sanitary annexe erected near the principal entrance. The guards provide a sentry for each of the three entrances to the grounds during the day. During the night the entrances were not guarded in any way', ends the report without in any way justifying this rather puzzling arrangement.

The first task for the augmented staff was to increase as rapidly as possible the number of beds, in preparation for the arrival of the wounded service men. This was done by clearing all of the commonrooms which the mental patients had enjoyed and installing beds in every available space. For instance the principal building, which in peace time had served as the hospital block of the asylum, had its accommodation increased from 150 to 250 beds and became the surgical headquarters with wards 7, 8, 9 and 10 adjacent to the administrative building; two further wards, 1 and 2 in the villas, were also made ready for surgical cases. Three operating theatres were available for use by the resident surgeons, who were later assisted by visiting specialists. Later two additional operating theatres, one 'magnificently lighted by means of a powerful electric incandescent lamp placed at the apex of a parabolic reflector generously lent by the Northern Lighthouse Board', were hurriedly opened in a temporary building erected to the north west of the administrative block which also contained anaesthetic and recovery rooms and more desperately needed ward space. Into the other six villas another 520 beds were crowded to accommodate medical patients. The sanatorium, with its two wards each of eight beds and its four separate single rooms was reserved for officers.

In under three weeks all of the alterations were complete and in the early hours of the morning of Sunday, 12 June 1915 the first ambulance train steamed in. Details of the one hundred casualties aboard were telegraphed to Bangour before the train left dockside at Southampton and by the time it was heard approaching down the line from Dechmont, Dr Keay and his staff were all prepared for the new arrivals.

Dr Keay later wrote the following very full report on the 'Transport of Sick and Wounded':

For the purposes of a war hospital the Bangour private railway was of the greatest value. Not only were coals, stores and equipment of various kinds delivered by the railway actually at the hospital, but the ambulance train with sick and wounded men came right into the grounds and drew up at Bangour Station platform. The removal of the patients from the trains to the wards was carried out by the Transport Company of the Edinburgh Branch of the British Red Cross Society, which provided a fleet of motor ambulances for the purposes of such work. The Edinburgh Company was assisted by the Bathgate, Broxburn and Uphall contingents of the same organisation. It is difficult to adequately express one's appreciation of the admirable work done by these men. They, with the ambulances, never failed to meet a convoy, and these nearly always arrived at night, from midnight on to about 3 or 4 o'clock in the morning, so that the Red Cross men had many a weary wait at Bangour Station on wet and stormy nights. They removed the stretcher cases from the trains, placed them in the ambulances, conveyed them to the wards to which they were allotted and actually lifted the men from the stretchers and laid them on the beds. They did this so efficienctly, carefully and tenderly for over 4 years that not one single mishap took place.

The cases in a convoy numbered from 50 to 300, according to the number of beds vacant. This number was telegraphed by us daily (at times when casualties were heavy twice a day) to Southampton and Dover, from each of which disembarkation ports telegraphic communication of the intention to despatch a convoy of so many cases was sent to us as an ambulance train was being loaded. On receipt of this telegram it was at once transmitted by telephone to the Red Cross Society's headquarters in Edinburgh so that transport arrangements might be made. Later on a second telegram was received by us from Dover or Southampton intimating the number of stretcher cases and of patients able to walk which the convoy contained. This information was also telephoned to the Red Cross so that the kind of transport required for the particular convoy should be known. Still later a third telegram was received by us, this one being despatched *en route* by the medical officer in charge of the ambulance train, giving further particulars as to the number and kind of cases of which the convoy consisted, such as the number of surgical cases lying down and the number able to travel sitting up; the number of medical cases lying down, and the number sitting up; the number of special cases, such as malaria or dysentry; the number of infectious cases, such as tuberculosis or influenza; the number of cases convalescing from infectious disease such as scarlet fever, diphtheria, measles, or cerebro spinal meningitis. On receipt of this third telegram we were in the position to have prepared the number of beds required in the different wards for which the patients were considered likely to be suitable.

The time occupied by the ambulance train on the journey from Southampton or Dover was from 12 to 14 hours. All the ambulance trains pass through Waverley Station, Edinburgh, and by arrangement with the officials in charge at Waverley, intimation that a convoy had left there on the final stage of its journey to the hospital was telephoned to Bangour Station. The receipt of this message was made known to the wards by three short blasts on the steam hooter at the power station and the sisters in charge of the wards were thus informed that the convoy of patients might be expected to begin to arrive in about half an hour. A further signal consisting of one short blast of the hooter intimated that the convoy had actually arrived, and that the unloading was immediately to begin.

Immediately on arrival of an ambulance train it was boarded by the Red Cross orderlies carrying stretchers. With the assistance of the RAMC orderlies of the staff of the train, and under the direction of the officer in charge of the train, these men carefully and expeditiously removed the lying down cases from their cots, placed them on the stretchers protected by blankets and carried them out of the train and into a large, well lighted and warm, temporary building of wood which had been erected on the platform for their reception. There, they were at once seen by hospital medical officers detailed for this duty, classified according to their disabilities, and ticketed for the wards into which they were to be received. They were then passed out of the reception shed by the doors opposite to those by which they had entered, placed in the motor ambulances waiting to receive them, and driven away to the wards to which they had been assigned. At each ward to which patients from the convoy were being sent there was a party of Red Cross orderlies, in charge of an NCO waiting to receive them. These men removed the stretchers from the wagons, carried them into the wards, lifted the patients off the stretchers and placed them on the beds, and then returned the stretchers to the empty wagons at the railway station to be used over again.

Another short blast of the steam whistle signalled that the train was unloaded, and that the last motor ambulance with patients was on its way to the wards. In this way with constant practice and experience, every man knew exactly what he had to do, and the smoothness and rapidity with which it would be accomplished was astonishing. Quite commonly an ambulance train with a convoy of from 150 to 250 cases was unloaded, the patients were in bed in the wards, the train had left on its way back to the port of disembarkment and the ambulance wagons had started on their return journey to Edinburgh within from $1\frac{1}{2}$ to 2 hours from the time of its arrival.

The transfer of the lying down cases within the grounds of the hospital and from ward to ward and to and from the operating theatres and radiological department etc, was carried out by War Department motor ambulances stationed at the hospital for this duty and some of those were driven by women.

The very first contingent of patients who arrived during the darkness of that warm June night in 1915 consisted of fifty-one surgical cases and forty-nine medical ones. According to a report which appeared in the following week's *Courier* the surgical patients consisted mostly of gunshot wounds while the medical patients were mostly suffering from the effects of gas. The *Courier* stated:

There are few serious cases and a large proportion are able to walk about the grounds. Clad in their hospital suits of blue the soldiers present a smart appearance albeit that the rather large turn up of the trousers, which is found necessary in most cases, does somewhat detract from the real sartorial effect and Tommy is conscious of it too. He seems happy, however, in his new surroundings and although life may be a little slow in such a secluded part of the country, he realises that for real recuperative qualities his new quarters could not be surpassed. Everything is being done by Dr Keay and his efficient staff to make the soldiers comfortable and already the nurses have earned the gratitude of the patients for their kindness and attention. Mrs Keay is also interesting herself in the welfare of the soldiers and is making an appeal for magazines etc, to help them while away the time. Writing paper, postcards and postage stamps will also be most acceptable and

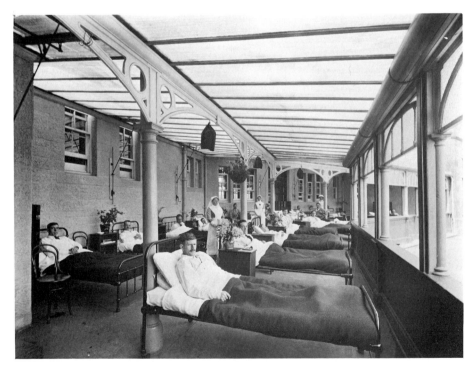

Fig. 7   Ward 2 Verandah where orthopaedic patients are drawn up with military precision—sitting to attention, eyes right!

can either be sent direct to Mrs Keay or handed into our Broxburn branch.

Our Broxburn representative called at the hospital this week and found the soldiers obviously enjoying their most congenial surroundings. Some were stretched out on the grass at the entrance to the grounds, basking in the brilliant sunshine. Others could be seen enjoying a quiet walk in the extensive grounds, while a number were seated in comfortable camp chairs. In the course of a conversation the 'Tommies' showed little inclination to speak of their doings.

During the following weeks more and more hospital trains arrived at Bangour, and the nurses were soon pleased to welcome the assistance of fifty V.A.D.s. One of these recruits who still remembers vividly her first impressions of work in the wards at Bangour Village, is 92-year-old Mrs Effie Day.

I had wanted to be a volunteer nurse from the day that war broke out in 1914, but had to wait until my eighteenth birthday. Although I was enthusiastic, I had absolutely no idea what awaited me at Bangour and what I saw on that first day made me want to run straight home to Edinburgh. I was told to take up duties in a medical ward but even there the suffering was terrible to see. There were young boys who had been blinded by mustard gas in the trenches in Belgium. Others were suffering from dysentry, malaria and even black water fever.

Officially I was a member of the day shift but hours did not matter. If an ambulance train came in we were all there until every single patient was cared for. Our shifts were so long that we all had to be resident. At first I lived in the nurses' home, which was very crowded with all the extra staff, but later I was fortunate to be one of the lucky ones to be accommodated in some cottages which were requisitioned for the duration in Dechmont.

Even when I lived in Dechmont life still revolved entirely around the happenings of my ward, Ward 24. I was issued with a uniform and the Matron insisted that my skirt must not be more than six inches off the ground so that officially the boys would not be tempted by so much as a glimpse of stocking, far less ankle. Although Matron was strict she was very fair. She had worked previously at Bangour when it was a mental hospital and knew well how to treat both patients and staff. I can never remember any friction. Everyone worked together and all the patients that could get up out of bed helped with little tasks to make our job easier around the ward. They were especially helpful when meals arrived. They were all cooked in the central kitchen in the grounds and were delivered in containers carried on horse drawn carts. The food was surprisingly good for the war years and the patients definitely ate better than the civilian population. As well as the main meals, of which haddock and chips was always a favourite, I also remember the lovely porridge with plenty of fresh creamy milk delivered fresh each morning from the Home Farm where a few of the mental patients were kept on through the war to help with the work.

As well as the main meals from the central kitchen, the ward also had its own little kitchen, where the kettle was always on the boil to make tea and no matter the nationality of the patients they all loved a cup of tea. Bangour was the first place where I ever saw a black man when we received several West Indian patients. They came from Jamaica and there were also many Canadians. The Canadians always seemed very rich to us, but as we were only paid £20 a year, perhaps that was not so surprising. We had one day a month off and sometimes I was so exhausted I just slept, but usually I travelled home to Edinburgh. Gas powered buses with huge balloons of gas on the roof ran once a day from the hospital main gate to Waverley Station and I was usually very sick on the journey. Whether this was travel sickness or the effects of the gas I never knew, but I often only got over it in time for the journey back which was just as bad. One week three of the Canadian soldiers heard that two of the other nurses and I were due our day off and insisted on taking us to Edinburgh by taxi. They treated us to a lovely meal in a restaurant overlooking Princes Street, but I could not enjoy it for feeling guilty about not going home to visit my parents.

On other occasions we went for picnics with the patients in the grounds and if we were off duty on Sunday evenings we accompanied them to the church service. We always prayed that the fighting would end and before our patients were well enough to return to the trenches. I promised to write to one young man, but although he wrote to me, with all the work and long hours in the ward I never replied. Months later his friend was carried in again on a stretcher from one of the ambulance trains and told me that the boy who had written had been killed in the trenches.

At last in 1918 the terrible war drew to an end and on the morning of 11th November the lady doctor in charge of our ward made the wonderful announcement that we had all prayed for.

The Armistice had been signed. We were at peace again. For a moment there was silence, then cheering the like of which I shall never forget. Soon we were all singing the songs that the war had made famous from 'It's a long way to Tipperary' to 'Pack up your troubles in your old kit bag'. Now we knew that none of our patients would have to face returning to the terrors of the trenches. Instead many of the boys went on to convalescent homes before returning home.

At last I too could go home, but my experiences as a V.A.D. had given me the desire to become a fully qualified nurse. There was a waiting list of 70 at Edinburgh Royal, but my minister, Dr Scroggie at the Charlotte Baptist Chapel managed to find a place for me at Sunderland Royal Infirmary. I went south and during my training met

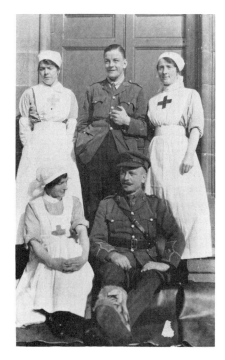 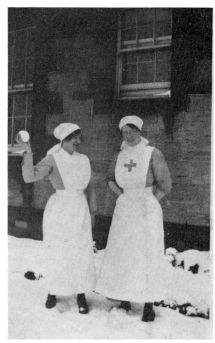

Figs. 8 and 9   Mrs Lilias Jean Durno writes:

> As a child I recall many a tale which started 'When I was at Bangour'. Such was the influence of Bangour on my young life that I also became a nurse and now my daughter, Mrs Dilip Meikle, nurses at Bangour and some day will say to her daughter—'When I was at Bangour'.

Nurse Mutch, the first of three generations of nurses from one family can be seen on the right of both pictures. The snowball fight in the second photo is a pleasant reminder that there was some fun during the bleakest days of the First World War. At the end of the war Nurse Mutch returned to her home in Fraserburgh, where she married her sweetheart W J Reid. She lived until April 1977.

my future husband. He worked in the colliery office near Durham and when I finished my course in 1924 I became a District Nurse working among the miners' families in the pit villages, but I will always remember my first introduction to nursing during the war years at Bangour, and how we always knew when the lads were beginning to recover when they started playing tricks on us. The long hours and the poor pay did not matter, we were all so proud of the job we did.

The very special atmosphere of these wartime years was also captured in a different way by one of the staff, who was quite an artist and drew a series of pastel cartoons depicting scenes in the wards and operating theatres. Many of them have been preserved and are on display in the Physician Superintendent's office, and some of the cartoons are reproduced on page 30.

The official records for the First World War period also reveal many interesting details of how Bangour coped with, what has remained ever since, its record capacity of over 3,000 patients which was reached in 1918. As the fighting had worsened so too had the number of casualties until by early in 1916 the wards and even the verandahs surrounding them were so crammed to capacity with beds that Dr Keay was forced to inform the authorities that Bangour could accept no more injured soldiers. Realising only too well that the terrible carnage was going to continue and that the number of wounded would grow, not lessen, the War Office, through Scottish Command, asked Dr Keay to come up with an urgent solution as to how the number of beds could be increased without delay from the existing 1,350 to 2,000.

Dr Keay replied that the existing central administration—water supply, drainage, steam and electricity generating plant, kitchen and other essential services—were sufficient to cope with the growth to 2,000 and suggested that the additional men be accommodated in wooden huts each large enough to house a complete ward of sixty. The War Office responded that there were no suitable large huts available, that there was no time to build them and that tents would therefore have to suffice. These tents were obtained from the Army Ordnance Stores at Stirling, which also supplied the necessary beds, bedding, lockers and bedside tables.

As soon as they arrived, the marquees—as they were always thereafter referred to—were erected quickly in close proximity to the existing wards to which they were to be attached for administrative purposes. The double roofed marquees were floored and each could accommodate twelve beds. Each was lit with electricity from the hospital's own generating station and heated by stoves burning anthracite coal. The marquees were utilised for the less seriously ill patients, whose wounds or disease did not prevent them from getting up and walking about. Fifty more beds were also squeezed into every possible available space in the villa wards despite their already overcrowded condition, but even after these desperate measures the total number of patients who could be accommodated still only reached 1,838.

With the hospital overflowing with patients the War Office decided that an extension on a vast scale was necessary and accepted Dr Keay's suggestion that the field to the west of Bangour Farm Steading be utilised for a complete tented hospital of a further 1,000 beds. In his report Dr Keay states:

> This involved a considerable amount of work. The site was laid out and fenced, roads, paths and drains were made and water and electricity current were introduced. A cook house of wood and corrugated iron with a concrete floor was erected and equipped with

boilers, roasting ovens, sinks etc. Adjoining this, stores for meat, bread and other provisions were fitted up. Other buildings of similar construction served as orderly room, dressings and massage rooms, bathrooms, ablution huts and a coal store. A very large wooden hut, with pantry annexed, was used as a mess room and the Hut Committee of the Episcopal Church in Scotland very kindly offered and erected a recreation hut with a dry canteen, which was a great boon.

The Camp Hospital was used for men with wounds or other disabilities of a less severe type who were able to walk and to some extent to attend to their own needs, but were unfit for discharge from hospital or for transfer to Red Cross Auxilliary Hospitals. Lieutenant Colonel J M Cadell, RAMC (late I.M.S.) was medical officer in charge and he was assisted in his surgical and medical duties by one of the resident medical officers and by a sister, masseuse and some nurses. Under the medical officer in charge, a Sergeant-Major (who was a patient) and an NCO of each marquee (also patients) looked after discipline and order.

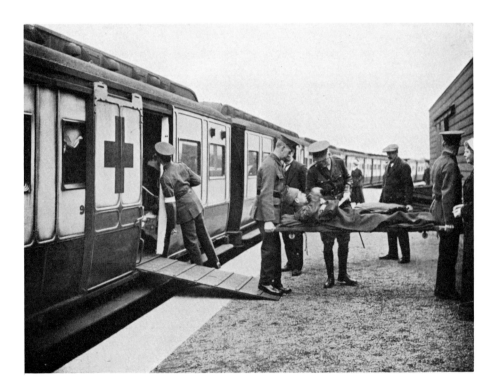

Fig. 10 A train arrives with a convoy of patients.

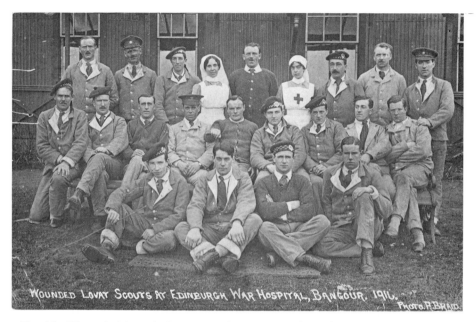

Fig. 11   Wounded Lovat's Scouts, having returned from Gallipoli, are still a long
way from home at the Edinburgh War Hospital in 1916. Courtesy of William Martin.

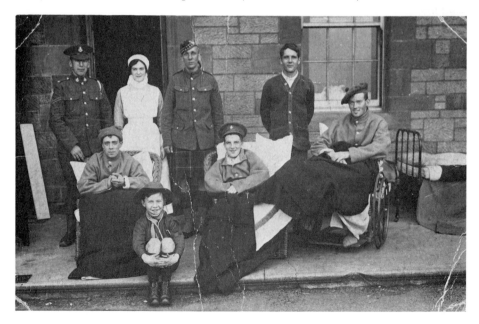

Fig. 12   A smart young Boy Scout poses proudly with Army casualties who are
wearing an interesting variety of uniforms.

When it was at its fullest in the autumn of 1918, the Camp Hospital had 1,198 patients and every single bed in the main hospital was also occupied giving Bangour a total of 3,036 patients. This amazing total was made up of 1,500 special military surgical cases, 800 general surgical, 496 general medical patients and 240 men suffering from tropical diseases and other infectious illnesses. Of the total, fifty-five were officers and the other 2,981 were all other ranks.

This enormous increase in the number of patients also put a great strain on Bangour's staff accommodation. The nurses home, which in peace time had housed eighty nurses who worked in the asylum, was occupied by 130, but this still left more than double that number without accommodation. The ten cottages in Dechmont, mentioned by Mrs Day, were lent by the District Board of Control as soon as they were complete, and were fitted out to provide homes for seventy staff, mainly on night duty, as their village setting provided a haven of rest away from the continual bustle of the main hospital. At the beginning of the war 105 patients from the asylum, whom Dr Keay described as 'quiet and useful', were retained to provide labour in the War Hospital. Sixty were male patients, whose help was much appreciated at a time when more and more men were unavailable because they were away fighting at the front. Twelve of the male patients were housed in the farm house and worked in the steading. The other forty-eight were accommodated in Home 23 and worked in the grounds and in the gardens. Forty-five women patients were housed in Industrial Home No. 18 and gave great service in the central kitchen and laundry, but as the demand for staff accommodation became more and more critical it was reluctantly decided that their help must be dispensed with and by the end of the war only thirty-eight male and twenty-four female mental patients were still working at Bangour. The two villas which they had earlier occupied were converted into auxilliary nurses homes, while the farm house was turned into comfortable, if rather crowded, accommodation for the resident junior doctors. Senior staff enjoyed the comparative luxury of Houston House which was requisitioned for the duration. At the start of the war Bangour's offshoot at Middleton Hall, Uphall, continued as an asylum with fifty-two patients but in the end the need for accommodation for Bangour staff meant that they had to be removed to other institutions, or sent home to relatives, or boarded out in the country. Middleton Hall then became the headquarters for the ever increasing numbers of masseuses needed to provide physical therapy for the wounded soldiers and in his report Dr Keay pays special tribute to the great work which these ladies did as sadly the war casualties provided them with more and more experience of working with amputees.

As in Northern Ireland today and in wars throughout history, the First World War provided considerable opportunities for advancements in medical skills and one area in which great progress was made at Bangour between

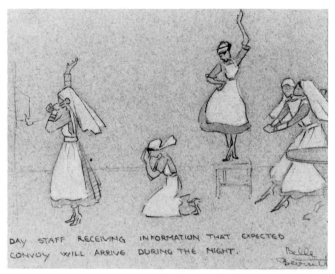

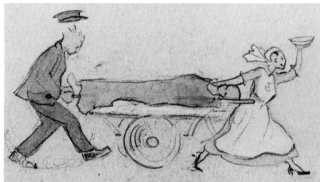

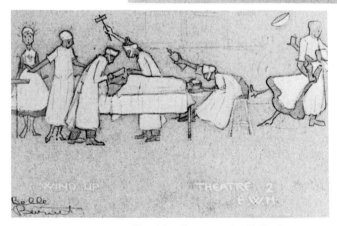

Fig. 13 Cartoons by Belle Barnet.

1914 and 1918 was the X-Ray department. The original asylum had a radiography department but it was contained in one room. At the start of the war the department was placed under the charge of a Mr Thomas Rankine who, according to a contemporary article,

> not only provided the whole apparatus, but generously placed his services at the entire disposal of the staff. Three rooms are allocated to the x-ray department: one large room where the photographs were taken, a smaller room with a large viewing desk with the necessary accommodation for preserving negatives and records and a dark room.

(By the end of the war the X-Ray department had proved so vital that it expanded to fill the whole of the recreation hall, and even more modern apparatus, gifted by the American Red Cross, was installed. Mr Rankine's original 'radiographic machine' was also American and, according to the report written at the time,

> comprised a 10 horse power motor and dynamo capable of delivering 15 K.V.A energy at the tube, a close core transformer with five steps of transformation from 25,000 and 100,000 volts, and a special arrangement for fluoroscopy, a trolley switchboard and an automatic time switch. This machine was selected after trial of seven other patterns, as the most powerful and efficient appratus obtainable. It delivers with ease 100 to 150 milliamperes at the tube, and enables exposures to be made in a fraction of a second if required. A portable x-ray apparatus was available for cases which require investigation and which cannot be sent from the ward to the X-Ray department.
>
> The routine work is almost entirely performed with a milliamperage of 50 to 100, which allows photographs of almost any part of the body to be obtained in one or two seconds, and almost entirely obviates the necessity for intensifying screens, with which, however, the hospital is adequately provided.
>
> An automatic timing device of special design ensures exactness of exposure of all intervals between one-sixtieth second and ten seconds.
>
> The screening stand is only employed in cardiac and intestinal cases, when it is desirable to observe movement.
>
> Radiography of the eye and orbit is performed by the Dixon localising apparatus which is a complete unit for this special work.
>
> Of the two large x-ray tables, one is fitted with an adjustable tube box beneath, and is arranged for screening over the table if required; it is also furnished with means for making rapid stereoscopic pictures with the patient above the lamp.

With the extension and development of the work of the hospital it was from time to time selected by the Army Council as the centre for important special departments. One of these was the department for Special Military or Orthopaedic Surgery, with Colonel Sir Harold Stiles at its head. The number of beds allotted to the department began at 500, but was gradually increased to 1,500. Colonel Stiles was assisted by teams of carefully chosen full-time resident assistant surgeons, among whom were, at one time, a dozen officers of the Medical Reserve Corp, United States Army. Extraordinarily good work was done in this department in bone grafting, nerve suturing, tendon transplantation, and other reparative surgical measures for restoring the usefulness of limbs disabled by gunshot wounds. To assist in the work of all orthopaedic wards a plaster and photographic department was established.

Then when cases of malaria and dysentery began to arrive in large numbers from East Africa, Gallipoli, Salonika or Palestine, Bangour became the centre in Scotland for tropical diseases under the care of Lieutenant Colonel D G Marshall (Major I.M.S. retired), Lecturer on Tropical Diseases at the University of Edinburgh. For this department five hundred beds were at one time reserved, and the number proved hardly sufficient. It was found that Bangour, with its elevated situation and bracing climate, was peculiarly suitable for malaria cases. The apparently most intractable quickly improved, and relapses were uncommon.

Later, when limbless men in ever-increasing numbers were being admitted and retained until their stumps were ready for the fitting of artificial limbs (when they were passed on to Queen Mary's Auxiliary Hospital at Roehampton), Bangour was selected as the Preparatory Hospital for Scotland and the four northern counties of England for amputation cases, with Lieutenant Colonel Charles W Cathcart in charge of the department. Two hundred beds were reserved for these cases, a number which proved so inadequate that limbless men in considerable numbers continually overflowed into wards other than those set apart for their accommodation. In connection with this department the making and fitting of temporary peg legs, and, in particular, of plaster pylons, was carried on at the Curative Workshops in a room fitted up for the purpose, and staffed by patients who were trained for this special work. The limbless men were fitted with their temporary legs, and were given time to become accustomed to the use of them, before being passed on to the fitting hospitals.

To relieve the pressure on Bangour, after treatment the soldiers who were on their way back to health were sent to recover at a number of convalescent homes which were linked with the hospital and worked in close collaboration with it. Organised and administered by the Eastern District Scottish Branch of the British Red Cross Society many of these auxiliary hospitals, as they were described, were housed in stately homes and country mansions taken over for the duration of the hostilities. They included Whitehall, Midlothian with one hundred beds; Wemyss Castle, Fife which could accommodate seventy; St George's, Edinburgh, twenty-six; St Leonard's, Edinburgh, fifty;

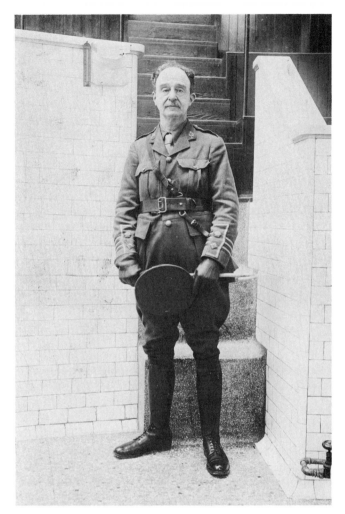

Fig. 14   Lieutenant-Colonel Charles W Cathcart.

March Hall, Edinburgh, thirty-eight; Cramond, Midlothian, twenty-three; Kingsknowe, Midlothian, thirty-four; Elie, Fife, twenty-five; Edenfield, Fife, twenty-four; Polkemmet, West Lothian, forty; Tillyrie, Kinross-shire, forty; The Gables, Gullane, eleven; Keir House, Dunblane, thirty-seven orthopaedic cases; Blair Castle, Blair Atholl, another thirty-seven orthopaedic patients and Edenhall, Musselburgh, Midlothian, which specialised in the rehabilitation of up to one hundred limbless ex-service men and fitted them with their artificial limbs. This gave a total of 655 convalescent beds available and by the time the war ended in November 1918 every one was filled.

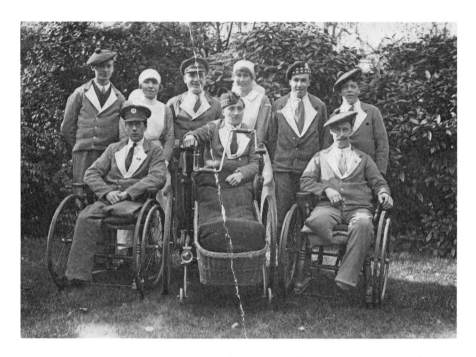

Fig. 15 The Edinburgh War Hospital gained a first class reputation for the rehabilitation of limbless casualties, as can be seen from this cheerful group posing in the hospital grounds with their nurses. Note that the basket woven wheelchair is fitted with driving lights.

Following the Armistice and throughout 1919 the 3,000 patients at Bangour were gradually reduced in number. First to be closed was the Camp Hospital in the farm field, then the marquees next to the permanent wards were slowly dismantled until all of the remaining patients were accommodated in the permanent buildings. The run down of the Edinburgh War Hospital and the return of Bangour to its peace time work as an asylum was delayed at this point, however, first by the reception of demobilised men and pensioners under an arrangement between the Ministry of Pensions and the army and, secondly, throughout September and October by a rail strike which made it impossible to return patients to their homes. Throughout the following year more and more men were either discharged or transferred to other military or Ministry of Pension Hospitals, until on 31 December, 1921 the career of the Edinburgh War Hospital came to an end.

Bangour's tremendous service during the First World War was not forgotten, however. Throughout the war years many West Lothian people supported Bangour by providing comforts for the soldiers including, according to Dr Keay,

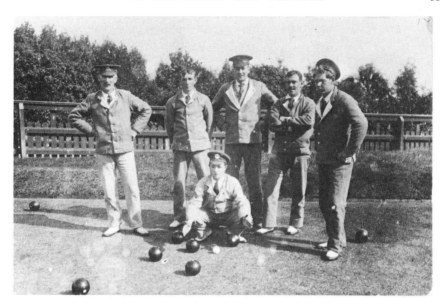

Fig. 16 All work and no play makes Jock a dull boy. The Bowling Club at the Village first came into use during the First World War and still flourishes in the 1990s.

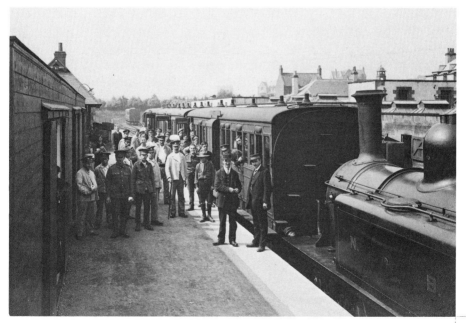

Fig. 17 A Job Well Done. A train departs with a contingent of patients being discharged from hospital.

socks, bed socks, slippers, dressing gowns, bed jackets, woollen
comforters, sleeping suits, walking sticks, cigarettes, tobacco, pipes,
flowers, fruit and vegetables, books, magazines, newspapers, writing
pads and stationery, stamps, playing cards, games of all kinds, billiard
tables, bagatelle boards, musical instruments, gramophones, musical
boxes, wheeled chairs, bath chairs, spinal carriages, a horse and two
ponies, the use of a pony carriage and harness, a motor car ambulance,
eggs, poultry, game, venison, wine and other articles of great variety,
all of which were gratefully received and duly acknowledged.

After the war many of these same friends of Bangour decided that Bangour's war time role should be commemorated by the building of the
beautiful war memorial church. Stone was brought from the Duke of Hamilton's recently demolished palace near Hamilton and the best stone masons in
Scotland were employed to build it. It was equipped with a fine pipe organ,
and with oak pews made by one of the asylum patients. It was completed
and officially opened in 1929, and since then has provided a place of peace
for both staff and patients. The inscription above the door reads, 'Friend this
House of God stands open for thee ever, that thou mayest enter—rest—
think—kneel and pray. Remember whence thou art and what must be thy
end. Remember us—then go thy way.'

From the outset Bangour Village Church was used for worship by all
denominations with initially the Parish minister from Ecclesmachan and the
Roman Catholic priest from Broxburn acting as voluntary chaplains and
conducting services every Sunday. It is only with the opening of the new St
John's Hospital at Howden, Livingston that a full time chaplain, Tom Crichton, has been appointed for the first time. As well as regular Sunday worship,
Bangour Village Church has been used on many occasions for the marriages
of both staff and patients and also for many baptisms. It has truly served
both the Bangour Village and Bangour General Hospitals well and is a fitting
war memorial to all who were connected with Bangour during the eventful
years of the First World War.

Chapter Three

A Haven of Peace

The re-opening of Bangour Village as a mental asylum was organised by Dr Keay in the same efficient manner with which he had run the War Hospital. From the moment Bangour was handed back by the War Office for civilian use on 1 January, 1922 arrangements for the return of the mental patients were handled almost like another military operation.

Dr Keay began by drawing up a list in order of priority of the buildings in the Village which required to be completely re-equipped or overhauled after their years of hard usage throughout the war. These included the power station, the laundry, the central kitchen, the admissions wards—which were to be used as Caring Houses through which all batches of returning patients would pass for assessment—two of the villas to be used as male and female observation wards and two of the industrial homes, one for men and the other for women. The Village Hospital's original operating theatre was also entirely re-equipped and provided with the most modern lighting system then available.

All the time that this was going on auction sales were also taking place regularly in the grounds as the War Office sold off the temporary wooden buildings which it had erected between 1915 and 1918. Again Dr Keay was active in persuading the Lunacy Board to bid for those which he considered would serve a purpose in his re-opened mental institution. Among those which he succeeded in acquiring were the recreation hut and two other smaller huts on the site of the Marquee Hospital, which he had converted to house a small colony of male mental patients. Another small group of male patients was later accommodated in the guard hut at the main entrance. The War Hospital Post Office was purchased and converted into a library to serve the Village while one of the best known buildings from the war period, the large ambulance shed which had been erected at the railway station for the reception of convoys of injured soldiers, was bought, dismantled and rebuilt at the farm as a steading.

Other problems which Dr Keay had to overcome quickly, ranged from the acquisition of a complete new wardrobe of clothes for each of the returning patients, to the appointment of clinical staff, both doctors and nurses, to supplement the nucleus who had remained to work at the War Hospital.

Dr Charles A Chrichlow from Melrose Mental Hospital was appointed as Senior Assistant Medical Officer—a figure who was to become a very familiar sight at Bangour during the following 30 years.

The speed with which all this was effected can perhaps best be judged from the fact that young Dr Chrichlow first drove into the Village Hospital grounds in his silver Lagonda on 28 August 1922, the very day that the first of the returning mental patients also arrived. They consisted of thirty-nine men and women who had been housed in asylums in Aberdeen and Elgin for the duration of the hostilities. Two days later a further forty-five former patients returned from Inverness, Kingseat and Banff. From then on every day or two more and more former patients came back until by 1 May 1923 the population of the Village Hospital had grown to 922. This total included several new patients, as direct admissions from Edinburgh had been restarted on 17 November 1922.

To cope with the rapid growth in patients Dr Lewis Paterson Foyer was appointed Second Assistant Medical Officer with Dr Susan A Binnie as Third Assistant and Pathologist. The spiritual needs of the patients were cared for by the appointment of the Rev W L Webster, Minister of the Parish of Bathgate, and of the Very Rev Canon Hoban of Broxburn as chaplains. Both held services regularly in the Recreation Hall as work on the fine new Village church with its war memorial chapel had only just begun.

While the 1920s saw the Village gain its church, this period also saw the end of its station and its railway of which it had previously been so proud. None of the former patients who came back to Bangour in 1922 were able to return by rail as they had departed, because, although the railway had served the hospital well during the original evacuation and had subsequently been invaluable throughout the hostilities for the transportation of wounded servicemen, it was decided in 1921 by the Lunacy Board that it would be impossibly costly to continue it in peace time. The little railway had in fact never been a paying proposition and even before 1914 the Board found itself having to pay around £1,000 every year to the North British Railway Company to make up the guarantee of £1,500 which had been promised by the Act of Parliament in 1900. The Act had set up an agreement between the Board and the North British for a period of 21 years and when it was discovered that the financial terms demanded by the railway company for a new agreement to operate the line would be even more expensive, it was decided by the Board to take up its option to close the service as from 31 July, 1921. The improvement which had taken place in road transport during the period of the war was demonstrated by the ease with which new motor buses coped with the return of the patients. Dr Keay noted in his report of

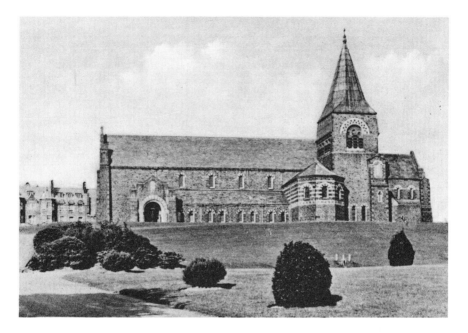

Fig. 18   Bangour Memorial Church.

1922 that even those who had had to travel from the farthest flung parts of Scotland had arrived without mishap.

Bangour Village Hospital returned quickly to peacetime routine, a fact noted by the Lunacy Commissioner James P Sturrock when he carried out an inspection on 22 December, 1922:

> The villas today were completely free from restlessness or excitement, despite the fact that very stormy weather prevented the patients from getting out. Indeed the only thing to disturb the quietude, even of the closed villas, was the haste of many patients to convey expressions of their gratitude at being able to return to Bangour, a sentiment which was endorsed by numerous patients of all types of mental disorder, to whom the return seems to have been a veritable homecoming.
>
> The dinner served during the visit consisted of soup, baked fish, potatoes and milk. It was a well cooked and appetising meal. The food is conveyed from the central kitchen by a motor van, which was seen on its rounds and inspected.
>
> The scheme of Bangour Village, apart from the work, entails for the heads of departments, especially Miss Davidson, who as matron, has charge of the whole institution, a very considerable amount of physical toil. It is learned that a daily visit to each department, merely to receive reports, occupies over 3 hours.

The duties and anxieties attendant upon the management of a large institution have been intensified during the period of reconstruction and re-admission. Under Dr Keay's able and kindly direction, difficulties of re-organisation have been skilfully and harmoniously adjusted. There are indications in the nursing arrangements, and the work of the staff among the patients, that the stress and experience of war conditions may beneficially influence this hospital, in the interest of those to whom care has again been so efficiently restored.

The biggest change which took place in Bangour during the 1920s was the admission for the first time of voluntary patients. This major change from the need for formal legal certification of all mental patients was first discussed at the Edinburgh Parish Council in 1925 when it agreed that 'suitable rate-aided cases should be admitted as voluntary patients'. This removed the former stigma of certification and, the necessary changes in the law having been effected, the first voluntary patients entered the wards at Bangour Village in 1926. By 1 January, 1928 there were thirty-eight voluntary patients, nineteen male and nineteen female, and during the following year, of the 343 patients admitted to Bangour, eighty-one, representing just under a quarter of all new cases, were voluntary.

In his report Dr Keay welcomed the change, noting that:

In mental as in physical ailments, the earlier proper treatment is obtained, the better the prospect of success. The great advantage of the voluntary admission of patients is that thereby treatment can be obtained at an early and probably curable stage of the illness, and, not only so, but the patient comes under treatment without the delay, the vexation, even the abhorrence involved in obtaining two medical certificates of insanity and the Sheriff's order before he can be placed under treatment, formalities from which many sensitive minds shrink until the malady has been confirmed.

The number of voluntary patients received is evidence of the usefulness of the procedure and fully justifies the Parish Council's action. In 1926 the number of voluntary patients admitted was 55, in 1927 it was 57 and in 1928 it was 81. It will be observed that 49 voluntary patients were discharged as recovered during the year, a recovery rate of 60 per cent. The recovery rate is really higher, as many leave the hospital when they are conscious of improvement, confident of the completion of their recovery at home. In case of voluntary patients a recovery rate higher than that which occurs in the case of certificated patients is to be expected. Their malady is more recent, they are willing to come and be treated, in fact desire it, and in the majority of instances the disease is curable.

While public attitudes towards mental illness generally improved during

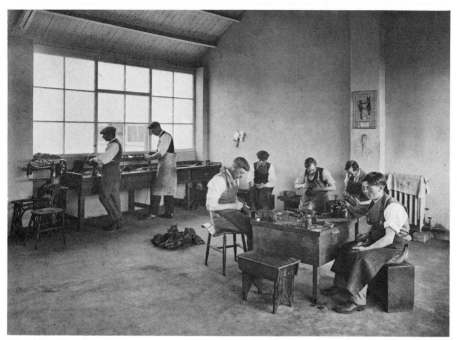

Fig. 19   The Curative Workshop where patients are making and repairing boots as part of their treatment as well as helping to ensure that the village is self-sufficient.

the 1920s there were still, sadly, apparently some members of the public who regarded those suffering from such illness as 'loonies' and a joke. This problem manifested itself at Bangour in one particular form in the weekly arrival every Sunday of local youths who sought their laughs at the expense of the young women patients, as Dr Keay explained in his annual report for 1928:

> During the whole period of the occupation of Bangour by patients the presence of members of the public in the Farm Road has been the source of worry and anxiety. This public highway is but little used for ordinary business purposes, but it is the resort especially on Sundays in summer, of people from the neighbouring villages, who come to satisfy an idle curiosity by watching the patients who are employed about the steading of the farm house, or who use the road when exercising. The farm house, occupied by patients, is actually on the road and, one of the houses, usually accommodating fifty female patients, is situated quite close to it. Parties of young men walk up and down the road, or sit at the roadside watching the patients, and refuse to move on when requested to do so. They have been observed laughing at peculiarities of conduct exhibited by the patients and

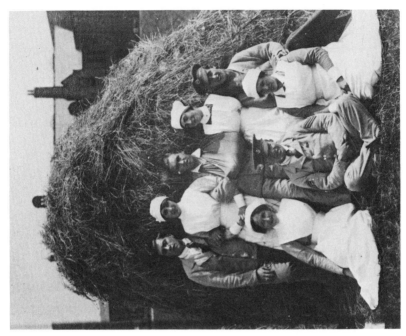

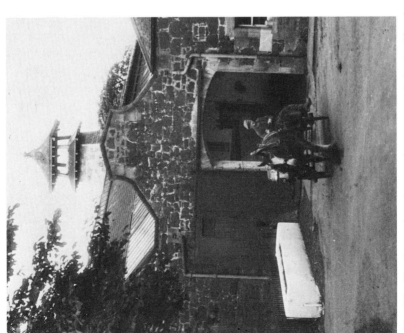

Fig. 20   The farm played a very important role in the life of the Bangour Hospitals, supplying produce and providing occupational therapy for the long-stay patients.

Fig. 21   Work on the Village farm had its more enjoyable moments after the hayfields had been cut.

endeavouring to engage them in conversation. On account of their presence the liberty of patients has necessarily been curtailed.

The public highway adjoins the buildings of the farm steading on three sides and these buildings and their precincts are invaded by strangers, who, when challenged, explain that they are 'just taking a walk'. Quite often they are found in the piggeries, byres or stables, and not seldom they are accompanied by their dogs. This is disturbing to the animals housed therein, especially to the cows in milk.

Having regard to the consideration set forth it is proposed that the Bents Road, which runs north and south at the western boundary of Bangour be reconstructed to meet modern requirements and should be placed on the list of highways as a substitute for the Bangour Farm Road, the use of which by the public should then be discontinued.

While Dr Keay was, in this case, eager to increase the distance between the public and his patients, he was apparently in many ways well ahead of his time in wanting to treat mental illness whenever possible within the community by the establishment of out-patient clinics and in the same annual report for 1928 he recommended that such clinics should be attached to general hospitals. According to Dr Keay:

The advantages of the association of such a clinic with a general or voluntary municipal hospital are obvious. Patients would attend more freely at the earliest stages of their illness than they would if the clinic were a separate unit or connected with the mental hospital; and they would have this advantage, that the ordinary methods of hospital investigation and treatment would be brought to bear at the earliest period of the illness, as in the case of diseases of other kinds. It is believed that through the operation of such a clinic, with a social services department attached, many sufferers would be restored to health, who would otherwise drift to certification and the mental hospital.

Part of Dr Keay's concern to see more community provision for the mentally ill no doubt arose from the continual annual increase in the number of admissions to Bangour, whose peacetime population of patients reached a record 1,001 on 31 December 1929. As the total number of beds available in the Village Hospital was 1,035 it is not surprising that Dr Keay looked forward with relief to the opening of the new mental hospital at Gogarburn, which was expected to take about 100 of Bangour's long-term patients.

Although Bangour had now grown to such an extent with over 1,000 patients, Dr Keay was at all times insistent that it must retain its family atmosphere and in this he was helped by his wife who played a very active role in the running of the Village Hospital, including taking charge of the library. Dr Keay was always keen to see conditions improved for the patient and one such case was his campaign for a recreation hut. He wrote:

Early to bed is the rule in the institution. The great majority of the
patients have been seen safely to bed by the day staff when the night
nurses come on duty at 8 o'clock. But there are patients, in particular
men, residing in the Industrial Homes, who by their good behaviour
and usefulness have earned the privilege of sitting up an hour or two
after the evening meal. These men are in twos and threes in the
different Homes and they would appreciate it very much if they could
resort in the winter evenings to spend a few hours in harmless
recreation. A hut is suggested, built of wood or brick, having two
rooms. In one of these there might be a billiard table and in the other
a wireless set, with comfortable chairs for those who wish to read and
small tables for cards and other games.

Dr Keay also took an interest in the patients' diet and was particularly
delighted when the board agreed to add to the equipment of the central
kitchen by purchasing a fish fryer.

The new fish fryer has now been installed [he wrote], and the
unanimous verdict of patients and staff leaves no doubt of its success.
The dinner of fish cooked by steam was unappetising, unpopular and
wasteful, a considerable portion of it going to the pigs. Fish cooked
in the fryer, and served with chips, is one of the most popular of
dinners, not a scrap of which is wasted. It is a pleasure to see how it
is appreciated.

Changes in the running of Bangour came about in 1929 when the Local
Government (Scotland) Act abolished all District Boards of Control and the
Village Hospital came under the control of the Edinburgh Corporation
Public Health Department. On a more personal level more changes followed
the next year, when in 1931 Dr Keay retired after twenty years as Superintendent. He was succeeded by Dr William McAlister, who equally became
a legend in his time.

The mental hospital which Dr McAlister inherited had a reputation for
being very progressive in its attitudes to both treatment and care. Bangour
always laid great emphasis on the range of its treatment from its hydro
therapy baths to its heat massage, and the 1932 report states, 'The resulting
benefit is not confined to the physical state of the patients for many of these
agents are powerful instruments of suggestion.' As Dr Alasdair A McKechnie,
the most recent Physician Superintendent of Bangour Village Hospital commented:

It has to be remembered that this was at a time before specific
treatments were available and most of the patients admitted, of whom
there was something like 300 a year, were in a very poor physical

state. It is easy to forget nowadays that the mortality and morbidity associated with the major psychoses was of a high order. It must be stressed that the hospital was designed originally for the management and treatment of patients presenting with major psychoses. The treatment of neurosis, whilst undertaken in some teaching hospital centres, was not seen as a major part of the service offered by psychiatric institutions.

While Bangour was modern in its outlook as far as dealing with patients was concerned it was still traditional enough in the 1930s to insist that nurses must resign if they marry. Bangour was recognised as a training school for nurses both by the General Nursing Council and the Royal Medico-Psychological Association. The course lasted for three years and was carried out by the medical officers who gave courses of lectures, the assistant matron who gave practical demonstrations, and the sisters who gave instruction in ward duties. During the course, nursing students sat two written examinations and there were also oral and practical tests.

Many of the nurses and other staff at Bangour at this time lived in Dechmont, a village created specifically by Edinburgh Corporation Public Health Committee for the accommodation of the hospital's staff.

Someone who remembers Dechmont well at this period is Mr Jim Thom of Laverock Park, Linlithgow, whose father was a nurse.

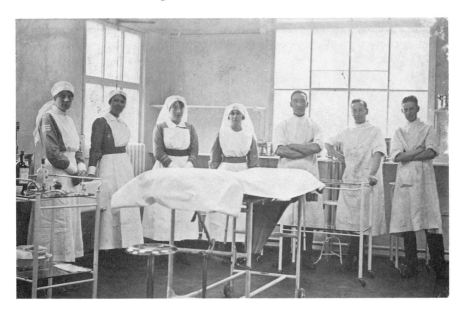

Fig. 22   A team of nurses and orderlies ready to start the day's work of changing dressings. This picture postcard is dated 12 May 1922.

Apart from the two roadman's cottages all of our neighbours had connections with Bangour. Not all of my friends' parents were nurses. Jobs ranged from butchers to bakers and from engineers to gardeners, all jobs necessary for the smooth running of a large hospital.

Names which still spring to mind include the Lannigans, Lambies, Burnetts, Gilchrists, Cockburns, Urquharts, Herons and Muirs. Robert Lambie, John McGuigan, Tom Chalmers, Hector Burnett and Roy Craig were all nurses like my father.

As children we had many contacts with the hospital. To get to Bangour we took the short cut along the old Mortuary Road. In summer we went to play in the cricket team. In winter a highlight in the dark nights was going to the recreation hall to see the black and white films which were shown there one evening every week. Another regular weekly trip was on Sundays to the beautiful Memorial Church, where eventually I sang in the choir.

The outbreak of the Second World War brought a lot of change and we frequently saw badly injured service men when they were well enough to walk along to the Post Office in Dechmont. Their visitors, from many parts of Britain, were often billeted with us in our homes as no other accommodation was available when they came to see their loved ones.

I remember in particular Mrs Sowerby and Mrs Sutton and especially Mrs Cleaver who came so often to visit her injured husband that she became known affectionately within my family as Wee Margaret.

The Cannon family ran the Post Office and were kept very busy with all the mail coming to and from the many patients for whom letters were the only link with home in those days before telephones were common.

Chapter Four

At War Again

The outbreak of war in September 1939 saw Bangour Village Hospital transformed, once again, into the Edinburgh War Hospital with the mental patients being evacuated mainly to Hartwood in Lanarkshire, Morningside, Melrose, Haddington and Rosslynlee. The government feared that the casualties from the expected German blitz would be so great that further emergency measures were deemed necessary and the Emergency Medical Service was quickly established to create thousands of extra beds in new temporary hospitals at Ballochmyle, Bridge of Earn, Killearn, Law, Peel, Raigmore and Stracathro. At the same time it was also decided to extend several existing hospitals, including Bangour Village, and so the Annexe as it was first known, rapidly took shape on its hilltop site to the northwest of the farm in 1940.

Edinburgh Corporation Public Health Committee minutes for 13 April 1939 records 'A letter from the Department of Health asking for an annexe of 1,400 beds to be erected forthwith.' A subsequent letter from the same department asked Edinburgh Corporation to continue to administer the whole hospital. Later the minute of 16 October 1939 notes the appointment of Mr Henry Wade and General Vere Hodge 'as surgeon and physician (part time)'. Later Miss Barbara H Renton was appointed as Matron for the 'duration of the hostilities'.

The 10th Annual Progress Report of Edinburgh Public Health Committee published in 1940 states, 'The [Village] Hospital has been adapted as a Base Hospital with 940 beds and the Department of Health are also erecting a hutted annexe in the vicinity of the farm.'

One of those who lived at the farm was Mrs Mary Gilchrist who recalls:

The tenants of the farm cottages heard with some trepidation rumours of a hospital to be built in the Covert Field. Would the children still be able to play rounders, football, cricket and tennis on the quiet roadway in front of the houses? Until then any vehicle, apart from the regular post, butcher and baker vans, were viewed with much speculation and comment. Would we now have a constant stream of builders' lorries, followed by fleets of ambulances? Was this a sure sign that war was imminent?

Rumours became reality as bulldozers moved in to dig out founda-
tions. One of the cottage boys became an apprentice bricklayer with
Arnott McLeod the builders. Would we lose the view of the Covert
Wood with its kaleidoscope of colours as the seasons changed?
Certainly we would never again see the Linlithgow and Stirlingshire
Hunt stream across the fields and surround the wood hoping for a
scent, then a chase. Fortunately the long low prefabricated buildings
hid little of the woodland glory, but seemed to nestle into its shelter.
As the war worsened the buildings were camouflaged and blended
even more into the background.

The minutes of Edinburgh Corporation Public Health Committee for
22 October 1940 state, 'Blocks in the annexe are now equipped, but not
occupied . . . they require heating and watching.' Ten stokers and two day
and two night watchmen were subsequently appointed and Mrs Gilchrist
recalls, 'The hordes of builders were replaced with maintenance men and
squads of cleaners. Then came the first of the nurses and doctors.'

Among the first of the nursing sisters appointed to the Annexe, in September 1940, was Sister Gilchrist, now Mrs M G Wade, who still has many
memories of these early days.

When I arrived at the Annexe there were no patients as the contractors
were still on site, building the five blocks, each consisting of eight
wards which were soon to become known as 'P', 'Q', 'R', 'S' and 'T'
blocks. Down in the main Bangour Military Hospital there were already
some patients, but how many and from where they came I have no
knowledge as we were separate units and only met up on social
occasions. The only link was Miss Campbell, who had been Matron
of the Village Hospital and who was then acting as Matron for the
whole Bangour Hospital Complex.
By the end of December 1940 we had a nucleus of staff at the
Annexe consisting of three Sisters and about six Red Cross nurses.
There were still no patients as equipment was still arriving and our
main occupation was allocating it to the appropriate blocks, preparing
beds and marking linen. The early months of 1941 were extremely
cold. The plan was that the wards were to be heated by three centre
ward coal fired stoves, which would have to be stoked regularly when
they were in use. But to the best of my knowledge they were never
lit, instead we, the staff, were provided with oil stoves which we
placed near to where we were working at the time. Extra woolies were
worn and our capes were rarely off our backs. There was a terrific
freeze-up over that period and so much damage was done to the
plumbing system of the newly built blocks that a central heating
system was installed with radiators and a coal fired stoke house on
each block for which a stoker was employed.
Sometime around the early spring of 1941 the first patients were

admitted to the Annexe, into Ward 1 of 'Q' block. They were not blitz victims or war casualties at all, but male surgical cases from West Lothian who were on the waiting list of the Edinburgh Royal Infirmary. They were originally mainly miners who required routine operations for hernia, haemorrhoids, hydroceles and varicose veins.

Another member of the original staff of the Annexe, who subsequently devoted the whole of his distinguished career to Bangour General Hospital and became one of the hospital's most affectionately remembered surgeons is Noel Gray.

I first arrived at Bangour in June 1940, acting as senior to two other Registrars, all three of us having been invited to join the Emergency Medical Service's staff by the Surgical Director, Sir Henry Wade. Initially I was not too keen to accept, but on hearing that some patients had been admitted to Bangour within one day after Dunkirk, I was persuaded to come north from Nottingham General Hospital. The summer and autumn of 1940 saw us occupied with treating the residue of the Dunkirk gun shot wounds, together with various other admissions from surrounding service stations such as Edinburgh Castle, Port Edgar Naval Station and the RAF at East Fortune and Turnhouse. At first these patients were all treated in the wards of the Village Hospital as the Annexe was still under construction. Meanwhile a number of senior nurses from the Edinburgh Royal Infirmary were transferred to staff units in the Village Hospital and they lived in the nurses' home behind the church. They lived there for over a year until the new nurses' home at 'K' block in the Annexe was ready, when they moved up the hill to become ward and theatre sisters.

It was hard to remember how my time was taken up in 1941 and over the subsequent years as a young surgeon, but from being a hospital solely dealing with service patients Bangour gradually became a combined civilian and service hospital because mercifully the tremendous number of civilian casualties which the government had anticipated never materialised and this gave the Scottish Secretary of State, Tom Johnston, the opportunity he had long wished for to improve hospital provision for Scotland's civilian population to a quite unprecedented extent.

What Mr Noel Gray means was explained by Tom Johnston himself in his memoirs when he wrote: 'I ticked off in my mind several things I was certain I could do even during a war. I had the ideas about hospitals which I was certain might be operated without legislation.'

Mr Johnston convinced the Cabinet that although casualties on the scale of the wounded from the trenches of the First World War had not yet occurred, they might yet arise in which case Scotland would be the ideal place in which to evacuate them. All of the time, however, he was earmarking these additional beds to make up the shortfall of hospital beds in Scotland and the resultant lengthy waiting lists which had worried and concerned him as a Socialist politician throughout the years of the depression in the 1930s.

Looking ahead Johnston was determined that, once in existence, the beds created in the wards of the Scottish Emergency Medical Service Hospitals would be retained when peace came to help the people of Scotland. However he could see no good reason why this should have to wait that long. He therefore set about persuading Sir Henry Wade, who had been appointed Surgical Director of the Emergency Medical Service, that so long as there were no blitz or battle casualties, it would do no harm and in fact would serve the country well to bend the rules slightly and admit some patients from the long waiting lists from the voluntary hospitals to the Emergency Medical Services Hospitals.

At first it was agreed that civilian patients at Bangour should be men from reserved occupations such as coal and shale mining, but Mr Johnston soon let it be known, very discreetly, that he would not object to women benefiting if beds were available and Mr Gray remembers well the first woman patient admitted as a result of a direct referral from a general practitioner.

The Medical Superintendent of Bangour Village, who by this time was Dr William McAlister assumed charge of all wards in both Bangour Village and the hutted Annexe and he saw his role as running a military hospital lasting strictly for the duration of hostilities with a view to him getting back to his work in the mental hospital as soon as possible. Dr McAlister was not at all keen on the admission of local civilians to the Annexe, but he accepted this as an inevitable development which would become standard practice in the post war period.

As Bangour was officially a military hospital Mr Gray recalls what he describes,

> As the rather anomalous position of having one's work inspected by senior Army and Naval officers including people like Brigadier Rowley Bristow and Brigadier William Anderson, who were concerned that civilians like me were being allowed to treat service personnel with serious injuries, albeit with the nominal support of Sir Henry Wade as Surgical Director. I recall a rather truculent Rowley Bristow arriving one day and asking to see any fractured femoral shafts under treatment. At the time there were four or five and he felt that they would be a good indicator of the general care being offered to surgical patients from the services. He departed in his staff car suitably re-assured.
>
> During the initial years of the General Hospital in the Annexe, the Edinburgh City Hospital divested itself of 150 long stay surgical TB cases and they occupied beds in 'R' block with TB spines, knees, shoulders etc. and genital urinary tuberculosis. They were all under

the charge of Mr Walter Mercer, whose lightning visits mostly, but not always, occurred once a week. As a result I seemed to be making plaster beds or other casts every week. I spent a lot of time arranging for the hospital joiner, who was more used to mending windows and floors, to fit wooden frames around these plaster beds.

During that time I personally operated on several spines, two shoulders and two knees while I assisted Mr Mercer at about two dozen others. Mr Mercer also had a plan, which never materialised, that a Thoracic Surgical Unit should be established in 'R' block and I assisted him at the first lobectomy for bronchiectasis to be carried out at Bangour.

Meanwhile more pioneering work was being carried out at Bangour by Professor Norman Dott. Norman Dott was born in Edinburgh in 1897 and was educated at George Heriot's School, immediately opposite the Royal Infirmary. He showed no particular interest in any form of medical career during his school days. Instead, when he left school, he was apprenticed first to a joiner and later to an engineer. A motor bike crash in 1913 led to him being admitted to hospital for treatment to an injured hip and it is said that, inspired by the surgeon who had operated on him, he decided to change his whole career and entered Edinburgh Medical School.

He qualified as MB, ChB, in 1919 and after holding junior residential appointments was, in 1923, appointed assistant surgeon to the Deaconess Hospital and to the Chalmers Hospital in Edinburgh. He early developed a special interest in neurological surgery. In 1923 a Rockefeller medical scholarship made it possible for him to study at the Peter Bent Brigham Hospital in Boston in USA, as a junior associate in neurological surgery and he enjoyed the inestimable privilege of working under the late Dr Harvey Cushing, the virtual founder of modern brain surgery.

On his return to Scotland Mr Dott built up a considerable consulting practice in neurological surgery in private nursing homes in Edinburgh, as well as being appointed surgeon to the Royal Hospital for Sick Children. In 1931 he was appointed neurological surgeon to the Edinburgh Royal Infirmary. On the outbreak of war in 1939 he was appointed Director of Neurology and Neurological Surgery for the Emergency Medical Service Hospitals for the duration of the war and he set up his famous unit in Ward 32 in Bangour Village and at a later date, a convalescent ward in the General Hospital or Annexe. Throughout the war and the immediate post war years Dott worked in the Village Hospital operating theatre and behind it he built an outhouse where he could use his original skills as a joiner and engineer to make surgical tools which still bear his famous name.

Professor Dott was greatly respected for all his dealings both with staff and patients at Bangour. One of the nurses on his convalescent ward, Ward 9, was Mary Bremner of Blackburn who recalls:

I had a great admiration for the late Professor Dott and his assistant Dr Alexander, who were on call day and night. I will never forget the day Sister was called away just before the Professor was about to make his rounds. Sister told me to take a pencil and paper and go round with him. I was a right 'rookie' and my legs turned to jelly as he walked in with all his followers. I need not have bothered, however, because he immediately put me completely at my ease. He had a great sense of humour and despite often suffering pain from his own hip injury he could always find time to laugh and joke with patients. I have many happy memories of my years at Bangour but none more so than when working for Professor Dott. He was a gentleman.

Professor Dott was also well known to the local police; as he continued to live in Edinburgh throughout the war his many high speed dashes to Bangour in his fawn or black Alvis saloons became quite famous. He also insisted that, despite war time restrictions and petrol shortages, a second car must be provided for use solely within the grounds of Bangour to transport his assistant up and down to Ward 9 in the Annexe and of course he got it.

Professor Dott continued to operate at Bangour until two years before his retirement in 1952, when in 1950 his dream of a totally integrated neurological unit was realised at Edinburgh's Western General Hospital.

Even during the war years Professor Dott had laid great stress in dealing with the 'whole' patient and was insistent on the best possible post operative care. He was among the first to recognise the skill and worth of the occupational therapist in rehabilitating his patients and this profession later honoured him by making him their Honorary President.

From the summer of 1941 the other blocks began to fill as Sister Gilchrist recalls.

The lower wards in 'S' block were taken over by the RAF, who staffed them with their own Nursing Sisters. 'T' block was opened as a facio-maxillary unit and Bangour proved an excellent location for these terribly disfigured airmen and both naval and merchant seamen, at a sensitive period in their treatment. The whole of 'R' block was taken over, lock stock and barrel, by the East Fortune Sanitorium under Professor Charles Cameron for the treatment of their pulmonary and spinal tuberculosis patients who all had to be evacuated when the RAF took over the hospital and established the East Lothian Headquarters of the RAF fighter command.

The East Fortune tuberculosis patients included many children and one of them who clearly remembers the convoy of ambulances which brought them to their new home at Bangour is Mr Robert Black. The move to Bangour changed his entire life, because he grew up in West Lothian, married here and still lives locally with his wife and family in Torphichen.

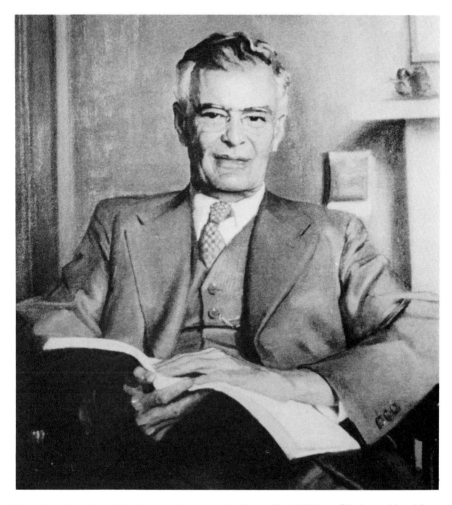

Fig. 23   Portrait of Professor Norman Dott by Sir William Oliphant Hutchison.
Courtesy of the Royal College of Surgeons of Edinburgh.

Five year old Robert became the first patient in Ward P7, an experience which he still vividly remembers.

I had TB spine and was in a plaster case which enveloped me from the soles of my feet right up to my shoulders. Most of the other patients were in the same condition and many of the nurses at East Fortune were convinced that we could never safely be moved, but the Consultant Physician, Professor Charles Cameron decided otherwise and ordered up a fleet of fifty ambulances to move all of us in one day.

As I had been in East Fortune since I was two I could not remember what it was like to travel in a vehicle and viewed the forthcoming journey as a great adventure. After I had been carried into the first ambulance, Professor Cameron clambered aboard and ordered the plaster to be taken off my chest. 'Now if you lean on your elbow you will be able to see the sea,' I remember him saying and I did and I saw not only the water but the fields and cows and streets and houses all for the very first time.

At Bangour I was carefully unloaded and carried into P7, the first of no fewer than three wards where I had the honour to be the very first patient. P7 was a mixed ward full of boys and girls all about my age and all like me, suffering from TB spines and TB hips. Like all the wards at Bangour, P7 had a verandah and during the summer months we spent all day and all night out there. In winter we still spent all day outside, but in the late afternoon the beds were trundled back into the ward for us to spend the night indoors.

The following year, 1942, Professor Cameron decided that I should have a spinal graft. The operation was a success but no sooner was it over than I caught chickenpox and so I was hurriedly moved to become the first patient in P5 so as to isolate me from the other youngsters, but it was too late and soon the others caught up with me. We were all therefore moved to Bangour Hospital's proper isolation ward for infectious diseases, R9, where again I was the first patient.

After I recovered from chickenpox it was decided that I was too old at the age of nine to share the ward with girls and so instead of returning me to P7 I was placed in P5 where I was soon joined by the other nine and ten year old boys.

We were delighted to have a ward to ourselves. During the day we had our own staff, but at night because I suppose of the war time shortages, our former nurses from P7 were still meant to keep an eye on us. Well, boys will be boys and we soon took advantage of this absence of supervision to get up to all kinds of tricks. After 'lights out' we knew roughly how long it would be before the first nurse on duty made her rounds again and that became our time for football. The boys who were able to get up moved the tables at either end of the ward into the middle to the passageway between the beds as goals and another boy and myself who were in body casts were positioned as the goalies. The others who had smaller casts slithered on their bottoms up and down the highly polished linoleum floor, using a make shift ball made from rolled up socks.

Night after night we got away with it until suddenly one evening just after 9 o'clock in walked Professor Cameron. There was utter consternation. It would have been bad enough being caught by the nurse but we never expected the Professor to walk in at that time of night. Without saying a single word he grabbed the plywood board chart off the end of one of our beds and spanked the lot of us. Not even I in my plaster case escaped my share of the punishment. As the usual part of my anatomy was not available for chastisement he duly boxed my ears. 'Do you think I've spent years putting you all right, just for you to undo all my good work in a minute,' he demanded. 'Don't let this happen again,' he declared and hung up the chart which had come in so useful and he stalked out of the ward.

It did not happen again but we still got up to plenty of other tricks. The ground at each end of the ward was cultivated in aid of the war effort with silage for cattle, corn, beans and, best of all, green peas. After lights out we used to persuade the boys who were up to sneak out and bring back loads of pea-pods so that we could all enjoy a midnight feast. Our basic hospital war time rations were also supplemented after most visiting hours which were from 2 to 4 o'clock every Wednesday, Saturday and Sunday. Each ward had a separate boiler house and usually the nurses very kindly heated up the tit bits which the visitors had brought in, but sadly we even took advantage of this. One of the 'up' boys, Geordie More, went out of bounds to the Hospital Farm where he found a dead rat in the hay barn. He succeeded in smuggling it back into P5 where, after showing it to us all, he wrapped it up beautifully in a newspaper. After the visiting hour as had so often happened in the past, he asked the nurse if she would heat up his fish supper. Her screams from the boiler house when she unwrapped it would have been heard down in the Village Hospital, but they were nothing compared to the yells of Geordie to whom she duly meted out his just deserts with the big ladle sized wooden spoon.

No doubt the modern child psychologist would be horrified to learn that Professor Cameron and the nurses administered corporal punishment to invalid children, but it didn't do any of us any harm and if any mother heard that her lad had been up to mischief and had been leathered for it, he then got another smack from her on visiting day.

I got into far more mischief after 1944 because a second operation allowed me to get up for the very first time. At the beginning of 1945 I was only allowed up for 1 hour a day but soon I was fitted with special callipers and a body brace and was more or less running wild. As one of the 'up' boys I was now expected after lights out to make tea for those still confined to bed. I'd never made tea in my life before so I simply added the tea leaves to cold water instead of boiling it on the three funnelled paraffin stove in the middle of the ward. The boys just about murdered me for wasting their precious tea allowance. I did better preparing our other bed time treat, boiled eggs. Each egg had to be held on a spoon under the hot water tap until it was cooked and I must have run off gallons and gallons of valuable boiling water but the eggs turned out a treat.

Our other after hours activity was listening to the wireless. The first wireless in P5 was a crystal set which we pinched from the girls in P7 but before long nearly every bed had its illicit wireless complete with earphone for beneath the blankets listening. Our favourite programme was the 15 minute long weekly 'Into Battle', which brought vivid descriptions of the successes of the allied forces. By then however we all knew very well that war was as much gore as glory as Bangour was beginning to fill up with seriously wounded servicemen. My saddest memory of all those war time years in Bangour came in 1944 when many of the soldiers wounded in the D Day landing were brought in. They included several who had been blinded and I'll never forget the ward concert when one of them sang, 'I can see the lights of home'. The nurses were all in tears.

As well as our own wounded soldiers Bangour also provided equally skilled care and treatment for a number of injured German and Italian prisoners of war and I was surprised how well they all got on together. They were certainly all equally kind to us, giving us sweets, which we otherwise scarcely ever saw because of the rationing and bringing into the wards jars of tadpoles, minnows and sticklebacks to keep us amused.

Our hospital school teacher, Miss Edith McMurray from Ramsay Terrace in Bathgate was not so amused with some of the ruder versions of well known war time songs which they taught us. Miss McMurray was a wonderfully kind and patient teacher who came round all of our beds in turn. For those of us who were fit to be up the end of ward P5 was partitioned off as a real class room, but even when we were able to go there our classes only lasted for three hours a day, which again left us with ample time to get up to plenty of mischief.

This included throwing what we called stingers around the ward. These were made from rolled up newspapers tied with string, with another piece of string dangling from them to which could be attached a comic or other article which we wanted to pass across the ward when we were supposed to be resting. We became deadly accurate.

We were also desperate to become equally accurate at billiards, but every time we sneaked into the tables which had been set up in 'R' block, the soldiers chased us. Denied this pleasure we spent more and more of our time going out of bounds. One day I even managed to walk all the way up to the reservoir at the top of the hill. I was accompanied by Geordie More, of dead rat fame, and we were just eyeing up the rowing boat on the shore when three gentlemen complete with fishing rods arrived and asked us if we would like to row them out. They even offered us sixpence each for our trouble, so although neither of us had been in a boat in our lives we leapt at the chance. 'Now the one thing you must be careful not to do is, if one of us gets a bite, to let the fish get under the boat,' were our orders as we pushed off from the bank. Well, of course, no sooner than one of them hooked a trout than that was exactly what happened and we were going round and round in circles. By the time we got them back ashore they were threatening to strangle the pair of us.

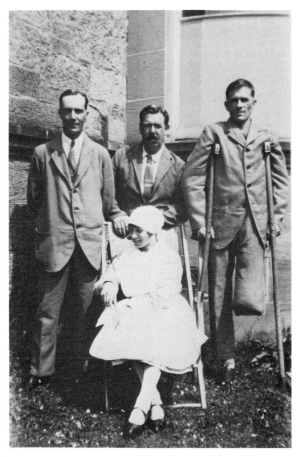

Fig. 24 A modest nurse surrounded by grateful and admiring patients.

That was one incident that we both got away with, but I really caught it over the episode of the cow. The other lads in P5 had never seen a cow so I boldly promised to bring them one up from the farm. This I did and if I had been content to let them see it through the ward window or from the verandah I might just have got away with it but I had a plan to keep the cow. Each ward had a brick air raid shelter built onto the end of it. The one attached to P5 had never been used as it was too difficult to move all of us in casts so it had been relegated into a seat store and now I decided that it should also be a cow shed. The other lads were thrilled at having a pet and we fed it handfuls of grass. All went well until half past one the following afternoon when one of the nurses went, as usual, to get extra seats out of the air raid shelter for our visitors. This time she got more than she bargained for because she immediately slipped on something unmentionable on the floor and of course a few moments later I got much more than I had bargained for from the big wooden spoon.

Towards the end of the war some people who did much to keep us occupied and out of trouble were the ward orderlies. We didn't know at that time that all these young men were conscientious objectors who were being made to work at Bangour because of their refusal to fight. As far as we were concerned however, they were all great guys. They organised a ward Olympic games at which even those who were totally bedridden were involved and awarded medals for the number of times they could stretch their arms. They also formed a Boy Scout Troup and taught us signalling using both semaphore and morse code and, of course, all about tying knots.

The Boy Scout Association can find no record of this Ward P5 Scout Troup, but its archives did reveal that Bangour had a wartime Brownie Pack. This was organised by Mrs Cadell of the House of Grange, midway between Bo'ness and Linlithgow. Up until the outbreak of war she was County Commissioner for the Girl Guides, a job which she reluctantly gave up at the outbreak of hostilities to concentrate on the war effort including organising the local Red Cross and Womens' Voluntary Service. When she heard all about the bedridden little girls in P7 she decided that no matter how ill they were, they must not be deprived of the excitement of belonging to the Brownies. She therefore, strictly unofficially, borrowed some of her meagre WVS wartime petrol allowance and each week motored over the Bathgate Hills to Bangour.

None of the little ones could get out of bed [she recalls], but the nurses were wonderful and before I arrived they had all beds already moved into a big circle. We even had an artificial camp fire made from light bulbs covered with red crepe paper and the girls learnt their songs and choruses and took their tests and won their badges just like any able bodied Brownie Pack. There was, however, one thing unique about our Bangour Brownies. There was one wee boy in the ward. For weeks he lay and watched all that we were doing and I could see the he was desperate to join in the fun. After one meeting I asked him quietly if he wanted to join and he agreed on condition that I never told anyone his name. The next week he was duly enrolled and became the only boy Brownie in Britain. If he reads this he will know who it was and that I have always kept his secret.

Another special happening every year at Bangour was Christmas and it is especially clearly recalled by another of the child patients, Mr James Harley, because of the role which his mother played in it one year. He was evacuated along with all the other child patients from Edinburgh City Hospital in 1942.

Our ward at Bangour, R3, was adopted by the officers and men of 603 City of Edinburgh Squadron, based at Turnhouse. These leather jacketed airmen were our heroes and as Christmas 1943 approached they promised us that we could have anything we liked to ask for as a present. I asked for a train set, expecting an electric or at least a clockwork one and on Christmas day when I unwrapped my parcel there was an L.M.S. train set but all made of wood which, of course, was not what I really wanted! Later however I became great friends with the Australian, Sergeant Laurie Mockford, who had carved it and although he couldn't produce an electric or clockwork railway, he somehow or other did manage to get a Partick Thistle Football strip for the boy in the next bed!

Something I did not appreciate so much were the wall murals which decorated the whole of the ward. They had been done especially by George Foster, a sailor from Port Edgar who was a patient in Bangour suffering from an injured ankle and he decorated the children's ward beautifully as his way of saying thank you for all the successful treatment he had received. All of his paintings were of nursery rhymes and fairy stories so, as a big boy of eight, I thought they were all very cissie and that we boys were very grown up!

I was much more thrilled when the end wall of the ward was turned into a temporary screen for one of the occasional film shows which I enjoyed so much. I remember especially seeing Bing Crosby and Bob Hope in *Road to Singapore*. It was at this point that my mother came in, because although we had seen some films we had never seen a real live show and she was determined that I and all of my friends in the ward should be taken to a pantomime as a very special Christmas treat. Somehow she managed to get tickets for us all to go and see Alex Findlay, the famous Scottish comedian, at the Theatre Royal in Edinburgh, which stood where the St James Centre is now at the top of Leith Walk. The hospital authorities said that they could not allow us to use ambulances because of the petrol shortages. Nothing daunted my mother immediately organised a fleet of taxis for us and the nurses who accompanied us. At the theatre we were lifted carefully in our heavy plaster casts into the best seats in the boxes overlooking the stage and Alex Findlay made a special point of mentioning the Bangour Bairns during the show. After the final curtain we thought that that was all the excitement over, but my mother had another treat in store for us. She had got together with the mother of another of the boys in the ward, Roy Walters. Mrs Walters worked in the New Cinema cafe in Princes Street and together they had arranged for us to have tea there with the police stopping all the traffic in Princes Street while we were carried in. What with the tea and the chocolates we shared with the nurses in the taxis on the way back to Bangour, we were all very sick the following day.

I had a twin brother who was very fit and he was always invited to the ward Christmas party. At Christmas the whole ward was beautifully decorated with holly, ivy and paper chains and one Christmas proved even more exciting than the others. When lying awake determined not to fall asleep before I discovered who Santa Claus really was, I realised suddenly that the decorations had caught fire. Fascinated I watched as the flames spread quickly along the paper chains from the electric light in the middle of the ward. Fortunately the alarm was quickly raised and the fire brigade arrived within minutes to put out the blaze. None of us was harmed, nor were the pillow cases full of presents which awaited us in the morning thanks to the enterprise of Sister Tait, who had written to the *Edinburgh Evening Dispatch*, appealing for toys. The readers responded magnificently and I understand that a total of sixteen big sacks of presents were received for distribution to my friends and myself on that wartime Christmas morning. As I was the only child in the whole of R7 who was fit to be up, I had the added thrill of going round all the other beds helping my ward mates, who were all in their heavy plaster casts, to unwrap their gifts. Hugh Nelson, Roy Walters, Duncan Hogg, George Renwick, George Doig, Andrew Gillies, Martin Dovey, Matthew Scotland—I still remember all their names and often wonder what became of them.

Once the novelty of all of our Christmas gifts had worn off we had to find other ways of keeping ourselves amused and wrote off for packets of stamps on approval, never realising that you were expected to buy and pay for them, until the hospital began to get threatening letters from all of the stamp firms and there was a great row. So we changed instead to writing to join the many newspaper clubs such as Rex Kingsley's famous football club in the *Sunday Mail*, but, as we never enclosed the required sixpence membership fee, we never received any replies.

We were, however, thrilled to have our own football star working as an orderly in the ward; he was called Stuart and played for Raith Rovers. Another male nurse, John, cut our hair by putting a bowl on our heads and cutting round the rim.

Every so often Mr Mercer, the surgeon, decided that it was time for me to have another operation. I remember on one occasion Sister Tait asked me what I would like to eat when I woke up. I said 'steak' although I had never had it in my life. When I came to after the anaesthetic had worn off, despite war time rationing, Sister had managed to get a real steak for me and how wonderful it tasted compared with the usual round sausages we got for breakfast and which we called 'rubber heels'.

Ward meals arrived by truck and once, when I was well enough, Mr Black the driver took me for a run around the other wards. Real food came on visiting days. As well as my mother travelling out from Edinburgh, my aunt used to come from Falkirk which sounded very far away in those days. She always brought home made scones and pancakes.

For six months I had to lie on my stomach, and then six months on my back. During the day my bed was pushed out onto the grass. I was supposed to be strapped in by my ankle but one day I fell out and shattered my knee. I suppose nowadays there would have been a great enquiry but during the war it was days before my mother even knew, and by then, they had operated and fused my knee leaving me with one leg several inches shorter than the other.

On another occasion I nearly killed myself. I was always a curious child and was fascinated by electricity and how it worked. To try and find out I got a 6 inch nail and stuck it into the power point behind my bed. I got quite a shock!

Fortunately during those long long days confined to bed we had our wonderful school teachers to keep us busy and occupied. Our headmistress was Mrs Gladys Hill who travelled out every day from Edinburgh. Her assistant was Miss Stobo. Miss Wilson also came once a month to give us music. When Miss Stobo retired she was succeeded by Miss Alexander from Lossiemouth. They were all excellent teachers and of course, being bedridden there was no way we could escape lessons or home work or ever play truant. The result was that I passed my Qualifying exam when I was only nine and later, when I eventually left Bangour and went back to school in Edinburgh, I was ordered to sit it all over again, as I was judged to have been too young.

After all those months in bed and more months when I was allowed to travel around the slippery slidey floor of the ward on my bottom, I still remember the thrill of being able to walk properly for the first time. Someone from Youngs of Forest Row, next door to the Royal Infirmary in Edinburgh, came out and measured me for a special caliper. I had then to wait six weeks for it to be made and fitted and then an even longer wait while it was adjusted but finally I was up and about. Even then I was so shaky on my legs I never walked across the little concrete bridge over the burn outside ward R1, I always slid across on my bottom!

For those of us who were up the air raid shelter at the end of the ward became our gang hut but even more exciting was the whole world outside. My favourite place was the farm and I remember once saving one of the sweets which the patients in the women's ward gave me. It was a red wine gum and I took it down to the farm to see if it would make the bull angry.

It is strange that James Harley from 'R' block and young Robert Black from East Fortune's P5 never met, because during the early months of 1945 he too was enjoying being able to be up and going down to the farm. In particular he recalls the rich creamy milk which the farm always provided.

It was delivered by a horse drawn cart, driven by Jim Dreaver. Jimmy Potter, who was one of the worthies from Old Bangour, who stayed on throughout the war as he was such a reliable worker, drove another cart which went round the hospital every day collecting waste food, or 'brock' as we called it, for delivery to the piggery. This waste was collected in what I recall looked like a 45 gallon drum on wheels, which was pulled by a small pony called Peggy. The boys in P5, on seeing Jimmy making his rounds, called out to each other 'here comes Jimmy and Peggy his mental pony'.

It was during the early months of 1945 that I travelled on a bus for the first time, saw a coal fire and thrill of thrills went to the cinema. All of these treats were arranged by the nurses in their time off. It was Nurse Skinner who took me to her home in Bathgate for tea and it was there that I first saw a real fire. My first bus trip was organised by the ward cleaner, Esther Hands from Uphall Station. Wearing my calipers and a special supportive waistcoat I managed to walk all the way to the road end and when the bus arrived very proudly paid the conductress the fares to Bathgate. The reason for the outing was to take me for the first time to the pictures. We went to the Pavilion, which is now a bingo hall, and saw *Gone with the Wind*! When we came out Esther took me for tea and I remember that I was so tired that I had to sit on the pavement in King Street while we waited for the bus back to Bangour.

I also remember all the kindness shown to me by the Sisters in P5 and P7, Sisters Maggie Barr and Mulvey. I believe a summer seat in Princes Street Gardens has been dedicated to the memory of Sister Mulvey. She well deserves it.

By the spring of 1945 we knew that the war was ending and one morning at the beginning of May there was great excitement when we were all told to gather round the wireless in the middle of the ward to listen to a very important announcement. 'This is London,' began the announcer and I couldn't resist shouting out, 'Aw is it.' Without a moment's hesitation Nurse Sneddon gave me a couple of skelps across my bottom and banished me to the air raid shelter so that I never yet heard Mr Churchill announce Victory in Europe.

Despite all my escapades and the well earned smackings that followed, I loved Bangour and all of the nurses and doctors who cared for me there. By the time peace was declared I was an orphan and I cried my heart out when it was decided that I was on the mend and must leave with a view to going to stay at the Trefoil School for Handicapped Children, which was at that time evacuated to Polkemmet House, the home of Lord and Lady Baillie, where the country park is now situated on the outskirts of Whitburn. They were very kind to me there, as were the staff of Wall House Childrens Home, Torphichen, where I later moved but I never forgot Bangour, it was my home as it was to my boyhood friends including Jackie Melville from North Berwick who was presented with the Cornwallis Award, the Boy Scout's equivalent of the VC, for bravery before he died. Others, who like me were lucky enough to survive were, Jimmy Brown who was nicknamed Horse, Billy Howden, Frankie Ryce, Robert 'Blackie' Knox from Gilmerton, Walter McGowan and Bert Guiney from Port Seaton. They all spent the whole of their childhood years as patients in Bangour. What became of them and where are they now?

Many adults also have memories of wartime Bangour, including the morale-boosting Royal visit by the Princes Royal in 1943. At that time Iona Gray, wife of surgeon Noel Gray, was a theatre sister and she recalls in particular the terrible shortages with which they had to work.

Even the swabs were washed, sterilised and used again. Hours and hours were taken up washing bandages and then carefully ironing them ready to be used again. Even our protective rubber gloves had to be repaired when they were worn through. This was done by cannibalising even more damaged gloves and then using them as patches to stick on just like using a bicycle repair kit.

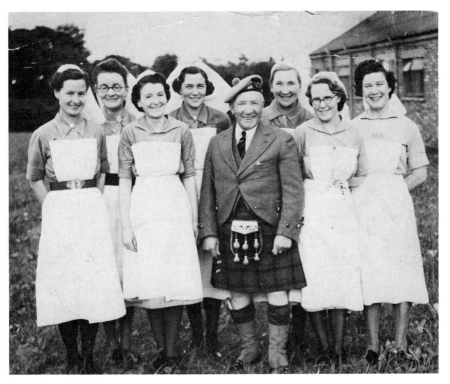

Fig. 25 The legendary Sir Harry Lauder was one of many famous Scottish entertainers who gave up their time to cheer up patients. (Sir Harry and this group of nurses are obviously enjoying each other's company.)

It was as a student in 1944 that Dr Jim McLelland first cycled out from Edinburgh to Bangour. He was accommodated temporarily in the Farm House and he remembers that the Friends Ambulance Unit manned by Quaker conscientous objectors, were resident in the adjacent cottage. Another member of staff at Bangour at this time was the brother of Eric Liddell, the Scottish Missionary, Rugby and Olympic athlete of 'Chariots of Fire' fame. Dr McLelland graduated in 1945 and returned to Bangour where his desire was to work alongside Professor Norman Dott.

Crichton Crichlow, the Assistant Administrator, had other ideas however and on my first day sent me up to the Annexe to assist Noel Gray in 'Q' block. I was also allocated accommodation in the Annexe which I did not like and, as soon as possible, made my way back to the Village Hospital where I was able to work with Dott.

He was a remarkable man possessed with extraordinary physical endurance despite the hip injury which dated from his motor cycling days in his youth and which had always caused him pain. He was as active at midnight as he was first thing in the morning. He insisted on the highest levels of patient care and this usually meant that there would be two sisters on duty in his wards and that the resident on duty actually slept in the ward.

On Mondays he carried out what he called his blitz when accompanied by all of his entourage, which included speech therapists, occupational therapist and physiotherapist as well as the usual doctors, nurses and students, he visited every patient and assessed their progress. He was a great believer in providing a carefully planned and integrated course of treatment for all his patients.

At Bangour he carried out his exceedingly complicated neurosurgical operations in a pair of hutted operating theatres situated in the Village Hospital. He also, however, had wards and operated at the Edinburgh Royal Infirmary and frequently rushed between the two hospitals.

On one occasion he told one of his ward sisters at Bangour to phone her opposite number at the Royal Infirmary to tell her that he was on his way. In those days phoning meant turning a handle and waiting for the operator at Bangour's manual exchange to answer and to put the call through to Edinburgh. The result was that Professor Dott was actually in the ward at the Royal Infirmary by the time the sister picked up her telephone to receive the message.

Traffic was much lighter in those days and it was reckoned that he could do the run from Bangour to the Infirmary in twelve minutes. Thirteen minutes was considered a slow run. His cars were immaculately maintained by Croal and Croal and when I accompanied him on these high speed journeys I always felt perfectly safe. He always joked that all I had to do was to keep my eyes open for traffic policemen! Although they must have known his fawn Alvis well he was never stopped and never had a single accident despite driving at over 100 miles per hour on every single trip.

In 1947 I was called up to do my National Service in the armed forces but immediately it was over, in 1949, I returned to Bangour before training in radiotherapy. I was appointed a Consultant in radiotherapy in 1957, a post which I held for 30 years, until my retiral in 1987. During those thirty years I continued to visit Bangour on a weekly basis, running an out-patient radiotherapy clinic for patients going into Edinburgh for their treatment.

Still more wartime memories are recalled by Mrs Mary Gilchrist of the Farm Cottages who writes:

Those patients able to be up and about soon became familiar figures to us locals and many friendships were made over countless cups of tea. The kettle was always on the boil despite the rationing. Outdoors in the better weather a favourite meeting place was 'Ham and Egg Corner'. This was the corner with the henruns on one side of the road and a field of pigs on the other.

Those of us who lived and worked on the farm knew that we were doing our bit for the war effort. Apart from the usual potatoes, vegetables, milk and eggs, we were able to supply at short notice chickens for special diets and very occasionally a small can of cream so that a hard pressed doctor's wife could add a touch of luxury to a meal for a visiting 'big wig'.

Now fifty years on one wonders what happened to all those fresh faced young doctors and nurses and their patients, who they so caringly and lovingly nursed back to health. Did the handsome Polish officers who looked as if they had just stepped out of a film set, return to their native land? Did the young airman, confined for years in a full length plaster cast return to his Highland home? I remember his young wife took a job on the farm to be near him. Did the Black Watch piper, who volunteered through sheer boredom to help pluck chickens, recall the hours of torture he suffered when hen lice got under his arm plaster and he couldn't get in to scratch them?

Although the hospital staff were always very discreet, stories of patients' bravery and the marvellous work of doctors and surgeons filtered through and the farm people were very proud of our hospital and of all the work which was done there.

Bangour's present Occupation Health Physician, former Broxburn GP, Dr Ian Thomson, also had close links with the Hospital during wartime:

The local units of the St Andrews Ambulance Association and Red Cross combined to form a single unit to provide First Aid Services as part of the Air Raid Precautions (ARP) units in the Uphall District.

My father, Dr Robert H Thomson MC, was lecturer to classes up to 150 strong. To keep the classes enthusiastic, training in home nursing was introduced. The men, mostly shale miners, under the late James Hume of Uphall and Sammy Maxwell, Uphall Station, formed a group of ambulance bearers, acquired a boiler suit uniform, and were on call to unload battle field patients from buses converted into ambulances. They would gather in Bangour Village Hospital early in the morning and await the arrival of buses from the Waverley Station. These wounded had been sent from the Dieppe or Normandy beaches, still in uniform, many with IV drips and in plaster of Paris to immobilise their limb wounds in the Trueta style of battle First Aid. The ambulance bearers had designed and rehearsed methods of stretcher bearing from bus to ward bed which was speedier and more efficient than standard drill. I was privileged to assist them and was most impressed by their gentleness in patient handling.

With the ward staff contacts made, these same men offered to assist in the ward nursing duties in their spare time. The civil nursing reserve was very short handed and welcomed the assistance in temperature recording, serving of meals, bedmaking and even giving the troops bed baths. After the end of the hostilities these men acted as nursing auxiliaries unpaid, for nearly two years.

Socially the mobile wounded were entertained in the surrounding towns and villages by concerts, dances and whist drives. A minor problem was the reaction of the good citizens unused to meeting severely handicapped or disfigured patients. A weekly dance was held in the Recreation Hall in Bangour Village. During the evening a consultant surgeon (N.A.G.) would pop his head in the door, study the dancers and on Monday morning certain patients would be listed R.T.U. (Return to Unit) having lost their limps in a Quick Step.

During University holidays I assisted as an unpaid ambulance worker, transporting patients from the general surgery and E.N.T. theatres in the hospital block–wards 4 and 5, to recover in their own ward.

In the emergency medical services annexe (later called the General Hospital), patients had to be wheeled from block to block for x-ray, on a wire stretcher mounted on bicycle tyre wheels—difficult to control especially when holding up a drip. Sister 'Frankie' Grant presided over Q3, the German POW ward—not the easiest of patients.

I became, in the absence of resident junior staff, more involved in ward work and gained a practical experience far ahead of my formal training in the Royal Infirmary.

As the military casualties feared, happily did not fill the hospital, civilians were admitted for treatment. I vividly recall an old man with prostate problems who was covered with 'paraffin warts', pigmented papillomata, due to contact with carcinogenic waxes in the Pumpherston Oil works. The lesions were so dense on his arms that taking blood samples was very difficult. In my student days 1942–1947 diphtheria almost disappeared. Penicillin was introduced. Later small-pox and polio would be controlled or eliminated.

As the general hospital built as a wartime temporary measure will soon be closed after nearly fifty years of service, perhaps we should remember that its layout was designed to reduce the number of staff and patient casualties in the event of bombs dropping on it. Thankfully no such raid ever took place and Bangour survived intact until the end of the hostilities in 1945.

Chapter Five

The Huts Are Here To Stay

Up until 1945, although Bangour was fully equipped and functioning as an acute hospital, there was no arrangement for the civilian population of West Lothian to be treated there. The time honoured arrangements continued for all acute illnesses developing in the local population to be dealt with at the Royal Infirmary or Western General or one of the other Edinburgh hospitals. General practitioners in West Lothian were not permitted to send cases direct to Bangour until the National Health Service came into being in 1948 and there were very few out patient clinics held until that time.

The first surgical out patient clinic at Bangour was organised by Mr Noel Gray in July 1946. It was held in the evenings in the Physiotherapy Department with no help other than the allocation of one very willing male nurse, Andy Patterson from Broxburn. The reason for holding this out patient clinic in the evening was that the government insisted that there was a man–power shortage at this time and that men could not afford to have time off work.

Opinions varied about the future role of Bangour Hospital and while Mr Gray and his colleagues all wanted to see it develop into a general hospital serving West Lothian and even further afield, the Superintendent Dr McAlister considered that it should revert entirely to its pre war role as an 800 bed psychiatric unit.

Mr Gray recalls one incident which helped force the issue.

Late one night an ambulance was racing to the Royal Infirmary in Edinburgh transporting a Bathgate housewife who was bleeding from a stomach ulcer. The ambulance turned off the A8 and came to the Annexe. The woman was bleeding badly and the ambulance driver feared that she would not survive the journey into the city. I agreed and phoned Dr McAlister at his home and told him that I would not be responsible for re-routing her to Edinburgh as I felt she required an immediate transfusion of blood. The patient was admitted and before long we had a whole ward of women surgical patients in 'Q' block.

Bangour had of course admitted women patients before and during the

68

war, but they had either been geriatric patients who were evacuated for a short time from the hospitals in the London area when the capital was threatened by the terrible 'V' bombs, or 'doodlebugs', or women from the services.

Sister Gilchrist recalls the service women well.

One day in 1942 two Women's Royal Army Corp girls turned up at Bangour. Up until that time there had been no accommodation allocated for women. These girls had active tuberculosis and so it was decided to allocate them to the isolation ward in 'R' block of which I was in charge. Soon the isolation ward was filled with army and RAF women recruits all of whom had active or suspected tuberculosis. By then the RAF was screening all of its entrants and some of these very young girls, who were hardly used to their new uniforms, were faced with traumas far worse than any wartime experience to say nothing of how to cope with worried and sometimes quite angry parents, who were determined not to accept the word 'tuberculosis', or even to discuss it. Tuberculosis was the great taboo of those times.

The service girls with tuberculosis or 'lung shadows' were soon afterwards allocated to other wards in 'R' block until they could be transferred to

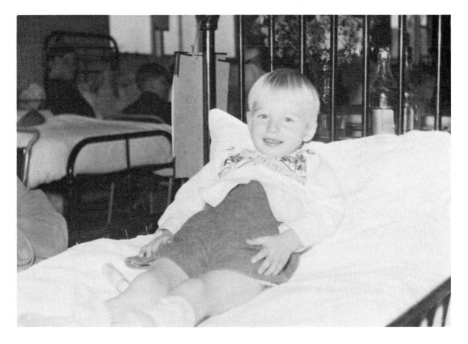

Fig. 26   Extra beds were also put in the middle of the surgical wards to accommodate children—young John McKail in Q3 with a broken leg.

sanatoria nearer their home, but by this time the civilian patients with tuberculosis were also being admitted and the beds were kept filled through-out the war. In the post war years tuberculosis was still the terrible scourge. In 1948 Dr George Summers was appointed to the staff and the tuberculosis unit occupied the whole of 'R' block where all aspects of the disease were treated. The Isolation block, then known as R9, was used for the treatment of tuberculous meningitis. In addition all the beds in Drumshoreland Hospital and most of Tippethill and Bo'ness Hospitals were included in this unit and were used for the less serious cases. In all, this added up to almost three hundred beds for tuberculosis cases and there was a waiting list of approxi-mately one hundred from the central belt of Scotland, extending as far west as Port Glasgow. This indicates the size of the problem at that time.

By 1966 the number of beds required in Bangour Hospital for tuberculosis was under fifty and the other hospitals in the group had become available for other long stay patients and the medical and nursing staff of the unit had now become increasingly concerned with the treatment of all forms of respiratory disease. Dr Summers' recalled:

> At first the only choice which we could offer patients was between medical care based on rest, fresh air and faith in God or surgical intervention. Six of my patients, including two women chose volun-tarily to live outdoors on the verandahs all year round. They were eventually cured and were in fact healthier than the people who came to visit them.
>
> Other patients followed a modified version of this course of treatment with compulsory periods of rest out on the verandahs every day.
>
> For patients for whom medical care provided no improvement surgery was the only other option. A favourite form was what we called 'pseudo surgery'. This involved injecting air into the pleural cavity to collapse one of the patient's lungs. This allowed the infected lung to rest for a period and hopefully cure itself. The treatment was repeated each week.

In 1948, as an experiment, four service patients were chosen to go to a sanatorium in Switzerland which, due to its healthy mountain air, was famed for its treatment of tuberculosis. They included Mr Leslie Nobbs, MBE, who recalls the experience.

> I became a patient in Bangour Annexe in November 1946. In these months immediately after the war with overcrowding, poor food and poor hygiene, by no stretch of the imagination could Bangour be described as a paradise on earth. A year later I had made little progress and wrote to my Member of Parliament asking him to investigate conditions. A War Office Investigation was set up. My morale was rock bottom at that time and I was therefore delighted and relieved to

be one of the four service patients chosen to go to Switzerland under the Don Suisse scheme. The treatment in Switzerland lasted 18 months.

It was during these same eighteen months that treatment of tuberculosis also improved dramatically as a result of the discovery of appropriate drugs. According to Dr Summers,

This was a big breakthrough in our fight against tuberculosis. The drugs available for the new chemotherapy regimes were Streptomycin which was injected and P.A.S. which was taken by mouth but which, unfortunately, had unpleasant side effects. The most effective treatment was when the two drugs were taken together but the patients were very reluctant to swallow the large P.A.S. capsules. Fortunately a little later Isoniasid became available and it did not have the same unpleasant side effect as P.A.S.

Using these new treatments the number of patients with tuberculosis of the lung was steadily reduced until by the mid 1960s there were only thirty and the former TB Unit developed into a fully fledged chest department.

In addition, however, Dr Summers also had to deal with many patients with TB affecting other parts of their bodies.

There are two types of tuberculosis, human and bovine. Cows infected with tuberculosis produced milk infected with the disease and this type of infection went into the patient's stomach before it spread. Before Tuberculin tested herds of dairy cattle were developed, bovine tuberculosis was sadly common and many operations were necessary. These were carried out at Bangour by surgeons from the Princess Margaret Rose Hospital in Edinburgh, led by the senior surgeon, Walter Mercer. We also had our own tuberculosis x-ray unit separate from the main x-ray department but under the general supervision of Bangour's well known radiologist, the late Dr Robert Saffley.

Mass radiography campaigns throughout Scotland began for the first time in 1957 when the first campaigns against smoking also began to take effect, especially amongst adolescents in whose age group tuberculosis had been a particularly virulent killer. Dr Summers recalls that at Bangour one of the very first members of staff to wage war on cigarettes was the surgeon Jock Milne. He neither smoked nor would he tolerate smoking amongst his patients.

Jock Milne was working at Edinburgh Royal Infirmary in 1947 when one of the surgical consultants suggested that he apply for the vacant post of surgical registrar at Bangour Hospital. He remembers thinking:

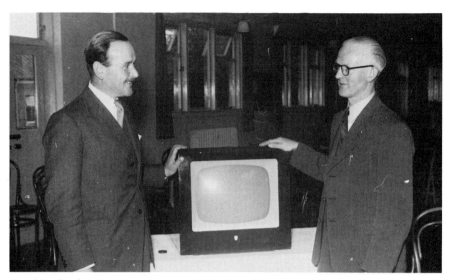

Fig. 27   Dr George Summers served Bangour Hospital and the many patients with tuberculosis and chest diseases who often spent long periods of time in hospital. Here Dr Summers (left) is accepting the gift of a television for one of the wards from ex-Provost Hunter of Bathgate.

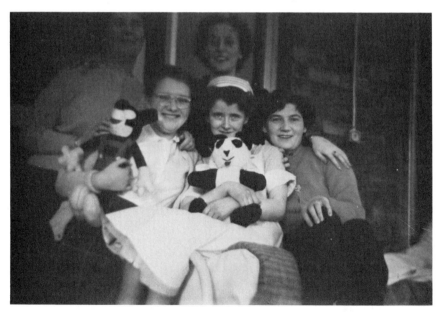

Fig. 28   Making soft toys kept the patients occupied, and, in the post-war austerity of the 1950s, were greatly appreciated by nursing staff, relatives and other visitors, especially for birthdays or at Christmas. A student nurse surrounded by tuberculosis patients and pandas in 'R' block.

Bangour? That's somewhere in the wilderness! That was Bangour as far as I was concerned until Mr Tammas Wilson, with whom I was working in the surgical out patients of the Royal Infirmary, suggested that I apply for the vacant post of surgical registrar at Bangour. The visiting Consultant at Bangour, Sir Henry Wade, was seeking a replacement for Noel Gray, who was going away temporarily into the armed forces. Mr Wilson also indicated that the post might well soon be upgraded to that of Consultant and, as an eager young man, I was immediately interested, no matter where Bangour was situated! The fact that in those days of post war accommodation shortages there was also a house with the job made it even more attractive. I had recently married and was now staying with my mother-in-law, having just come back from a period of overseas service with the army for four years. My mind was easily made up. My last remaining worry was the prospect of Noel Gray's return but I was assured that as a District Hospital and with the coming of the new National Health Service, there would be ample opportunity for both of us, and so it turned out to be.

From the outset I found that Bangour offered the kind of opportunities which my contemporaries in the Edinburgh hospitals could only dream about. They were hide bound by traditional practices. Bangour had no traditions and there was such a tiny staff that I could turn my hand to anything I fancied in the widest possible scope of general surgical practice. Like my own, Sir Henry Wade's family were of farming stock and I think this gave us a certain common bond. He certainly placed a great deal of trust in me and even when I went off two or three afternoons every week to lecture in anatomy, physiology and pathology at Edinburgh University no questions were asked. My former colleagues in Edinburgh were amazed and, I think, even a little envious, at my freedom and opportunities and were even more surprised when I was able to take a month's leave to visit St Mark's Hospital in London to study the wonderful colo-rectal surgery being done there by the great Mr Gabriel. His book on the subject was the 'Bible' as far as I was concerned and I learned much, but was still very anxious when I returned to Bangour about to perform my first major elective bowel operation and partial gastrectomy. Although I had done four years of emergency surgery during the war, I hadn't done much elective surgery.

I like to think of us who worked at Bangour in those early days of the General Hospital as the last of the few truly general surgeons. Walter Mercer was not just a great orthopaedic surgeon but was every bit as capable in his work in chest surgery as when operating on the rectum. Norman Dott also had this same gift of versatility in neurosurgery and yet he was the most humble of men. He would start to operate at 5 a.m. and was so patient and meticulous that for fourteen or even eighteen hours he would work despite any pain which he himself might be feeling in the leg which he injured in a motor cycle accident, and on which Sir Henry Wade had operated.

Before the motor cycle accident Professor Dott had served an apprenticeship as an engineer and when he was at Bangour he still made many of his own instruments and the little refinements which he perfected have made Dott's scalpels and Dott's retractors world famous.

Tommy Millar, Honorary Consultant Surgeon at that time, visited Bangour weekly to conduct his ward rounds having been the resident consultant surgeon during the war.

All this time Bangour was expanding. A new x-ray department was opened in 'Q' block which was surgical, 'P' block was medical, 'R' block was still the East Fortune tuberculosis unit, 'S' block became the maternity unit and 'T' block was burns and plastic surgery. Despite this growth, Bangour managed to retain its family atmosphere and we aimed to provide all the treatment which the people of West Lothian required. For instance, when we started our first out patient clinics, something so very much taken for granted nowadays, all the appointments were made in the evening from 7 p.m. onwards so as not to take men away from their day time work and the post war effort. Later when we opened the new surgical out patients department, Sister Higgins was in charge and finally we opened an accident and emergency department run by Sister Sanderson.

That first out patient clinic was held down in the occupational therapy hall at Bangour Village Hospital and it was very much a 'do it yourself' affair. We didn't even have a secretary and there was nowhere for the patients to change. The only help which we had was from a well known male nurse Andy Patterson.

Andy was one of the marvellous characters with whom Bangour was blessed in the early years. I also recall Sister Christie who came from service in the Royal Navy and continued at Bangour for 35 years until she finally retired to Ballachullish. She was one of my ward sisters along with Sister Grant, Sister Allan and Sister Wade. During the war there was also Sister Iona Macleod who later became Mrs Noel Gray.

At first, as I mentioned earlier, I lived in the house in the grounds which came with my first post. The fact that so many of us lived in, and so few had cars, meant that there was a great community spirit about the place and this included everyone not just the medical staff. Other members of staff living in the flats included Tommy Chalmers later to become consultant surgeon in Dunfermline and West Fife and Donald Irving, consultant obstetrician and gynaecologist in Edinburgh.

In summer we played tennis and cricket with the head gardener, Mr Thirkell—a Yorkshireman—as Captain of the Bangour Cricket Team. In winter we organised bridge matches and regular Scottish Country Dances. Everyone looked forward to the dances in the Recreation Hall;

store keepers, doctors, secretaries and nurses all took the floor to the music of Tim Wright and his Broadcasting Band. On Sundays we all attended services in the Memorial Church conducted first by Mr Pinkerton and then by Mr Edmund, the minister at Ecclesmachan Kirk.

In 1956 we moved to live at Craigbinning, Dechmont where my son Robert, who is a general practitioner in Kirkliston, and his family still live. My two daughters were at school in Edinburgh but could not wait each afternoon to get home to play with their pet dog, a spaniel called Texas. One evening when I got home they were most upset because Texas was ill. I promised to take him to the vet next morning and so I bundled him into the car when I set off for the hospital. After a quick check that all was well at Bangour, I drove over to the vet at Midcalder. After the vet had seen to Texas and kept him, I motored back along the country roads which are now in the heart of Livingston and thought about the huge expansion which was about to take place and how it would inevitably affect us at Bangour and the services we had to provide.

That was the last thing I remember for quite some time because at a crossroads my car was hit by a lorry. Looking back it seems quite ironic, because only a few days earlier I had been filmed in my 'greens' in the operating theatre for a television programme which Scottish Television was making about the dangers of the Killer A8, and some years before the new motorway was constructed, I had warned drivers about how very careful they must be.

Now I had the opportunity to find out how well Bangour looked after the many road casualties who were carried in to the accident and emergency department. Although I knew nothing about it at the time, an ambulance was on standby to rush me into the Edinburgh Royal Infirmary, but my colleague Noel Gray rightly determined that I would never survive the journey and that my only hope was for him to operate straight away.

I had a ruptured spleen, a ruptured diaphragm, every rib was broken and I had head injuries, but thanks to his skill and that of the theatre team I survived. After a long session in theatre I was taken to my own ward where Sister Christie and her nurses were waiting. Along with Noel, Sister Christie sat up all night at my bedside. My condition slowly improved and, agreeing with me that the most dangerous thing for patients is bed because of the danger of thrombosis, they wasted as little time as possible in getting me up but I was six weeks in the ward and a lot longer before I was really back on my feet.

My experience of being a patient in my own hospital was a valuable one, as it helped me to appreciate all the more just how much care we all need when we are ill. I often wished that I could have spent more time with patients getting to know the minutest details of their medical history before contemplating surgery. All surgeons should do their homework before reaching for the knife. My motto was always 'Don't use the knife unless you have to', and I was well known for my theory that many illnesses were self-inflicted and that patients could avoid many of their troubles if they would only change their life styles.

I operated on over 1,200 stomachs mainly for duodenal ulcers caused by smoking and stress. A number of my patients suffered from obesity and I felt so strongly about such matters it is hardly surprising that my ward rounds became somewhat famous because I felt I had a duty to be honest with patients and explain that I could not operate unless they lost some weight. The main reason for our Scottish weight problem is that even today we have a 'sweet tooth' and there were occasions when I raided a few patients lockers and confiscated the biscuits and sweeties. In time my view became so well known that I'm sure that my patients knew what was coming. I felt equally strongly about smoking and banned my patients from having cigarettes in the wards.

Over the years I saw many improvements at Bangour; better theatre and operating techniques meant patients suffered from fewer infections and allowed us to achieve a higher turn over of patients. I also enjoyed teaching the ever increasing number of students who came to learn at Bangour. They included Tony Gunn, who was eventually to become a valued colleague and Bill Taylor who is now a professor of surgery in Sheffield.

I was not so fond of the ever increasing red tape and bureaucracy. After the coming of the National Health Service Bangour General Hospital continued to run smoothly under its local board of management, with fine service from people like the Chairman Jimmy Kidd and Mr Crighton. Then, in the 1960s, the administrative structure began to grow rapidly and as the years passed we suffered from a decided surfeit of reports and management changes. The Salmon Report on the deployment of nurses was, in my opinion, one of the worst, as it helped take good nurses out of the wards where they were most needed.

I have many happy memories of Bangour right up until my retirement in December 1975. My family grew up there and many people still speak about the driverless car coming through the fields which was really one of the Milne boys at the wheel taking his injured brother to casualty long before he could drive on the open road. I thought that I too was sometimes at the wheel in Bangour during some of its most interesting years and may have helped steer it on its course as a hospital which truly related to its patients and their needs.

'What a dreadful, dreary place!' That was Dr Joyce Grainger's initial reaction to a first brief glimpse of Bangour Annexe in 1947 when, as a resident house officer at Law Hospital near Carluke, she went to collect the new 'wonder drug' Streptomycin which had recently become available for the treatment of tuberculosis:

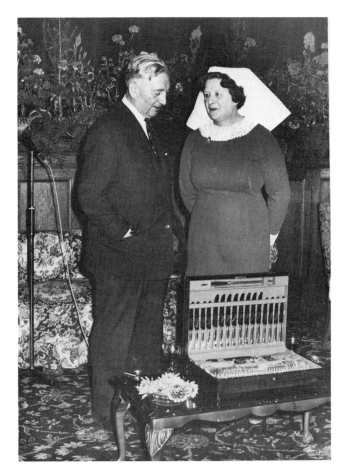

Fig. 29 Lieutenant-Colonel J Kidd was Chairman of the Hospital Board of Management in West Lothian for many years. One of the many happy duties he carried out was to make a presentation to Miss M Morrison on her retirement from the post of Matron to Bangour Village Hospital on 1 October 1968.

It was a wet, miserable day when I drove up the hill and caught my first sight of the sprawl of the Annexe. The only word which could adequately describe the scene was the old Scottish one—driech—and I remember thinking how glad I was not to be working there.

Dr Grainger was, however, keen to return to her home in Edinburgh and when the post of medical registrar became vacant at Bangour some time later she applied and was appointed to the vacancy in 1949.

On my first night I thought it unlikely I would last out a year at Bangour and was appalled to learn that one member of the staff who was a junior hospital medical officer in the Chest and Tuberculosis Unit had already been there for about 10 years. The appointment that I held was for two years in the first instance and I certainly never guessed that I was eventually going to remain at Bangour for 33 years!

Although one of Dr Grainger's reasons for applying for the post was to be near Edinburgh, she was not at that time allowed to live at home as her contract dictated that she must be resident.

Some of the resident medical staff actually enjoyed living in and at that time none of the junior staff were married or had family commitments. There were certainly amusing episodes but on the whole I found it tedious, rather like living in a boarding school. The bedrooms were tiny with scarcely room to sit and the sitting rooms were even less attractive with a collection of shabby old armchairs and little else. There was also a sort of library with a radio. After six months I was given permission to live at home and was glad to move out of the residency.

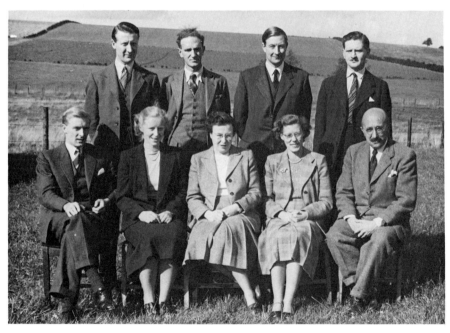

Fig. 30   The nine resident medical staff of 1951, photographed against a rural background in marked contrast to the usual more formal setting in a city hospital. *Rear:* Dr F Innes, Dr W Bell, Dr H Thomas, Dr D Maclean. *Front:* Dr Frickley, Dr A Sutherland, Dr J Grainger, Dr J Worling, Dr Buchan.

Dr Grainger has many memories of the staff in those early days at Bangour including Dr Alastair Wright, consultant physician, and Jock, the porter, to whom everyone was 'son or lass' no matter where they worked.

We had a very small staff compared with today and always seemed to be working and, although I was living at home, I spent all my time at Bangour with practically no time off duty. To begin with there were only two medical wards situated in Q7 and Q8, each officially with twenty-eight beds and often more. The hospital was smaller and all the staff knew one another. I well remember the Pharmacy which was a funny little place with a pharmacist who would only dispense a limited number of routine medicines and woe betide anyone who tried to obtain something that was not frequently used.

Dr Ella Purdie was the bacteriologist and Jimmy Tait was the senior technician in Haematology. Mr Bob Whytock was also a senior laboratory technician, working in Bacteriology.

Other names and faces from the early 1950s which come to mind include my predecessor David Ellison, and Margaret Addly who was house physician in the TB Unit and who had previously worked in the medical unit. Dr Ranald Murray-Lyon was the visiting physician and he did a ward round on Thursday afternoons. One cannot forget Sister Chisholm who came from Beauly. She was a character indeed and ruled the male ward and its staff with a rod of iron. Her staff nurse was known as 'Young Chris' to those of us in the medical unit but when she moved to the gynaecology department she then became Sister McDonald. Sister Chisholm was later succeeded by Effie Maclean. On the female side Sister Gibson was followed by Nan Grieve who is now Chief Nursing Officer in the Central Region of Scotland, based at Stirling.

As well as professional duties Dr Grainger recalls the social life for which Bangour was well known in those days.

The recreation hall in the Village Hospital was the centre for social activities and the Annual Christmas Party for the staff was held there. We all attended in the certain knowledge that there would be no alcohol served as the Superintendent, Dr Willie McAlister was strictly 'tee-total'. Fortunately Donald Irving, who was at that time a senior obstetric registrar, had a house in the grounds of the General Hospital and we were generously entertained by Donald and his wife before the party. I do remember one occasion when Paddy Aitcheson, one of our house surgeons, managed to add some gin to the orange squash on the tables.

To the junior staff, Dr McAlister was remote and austere in his manner. Miss Campbell, the Matron of the Village Hospital was, however, most hospitable.

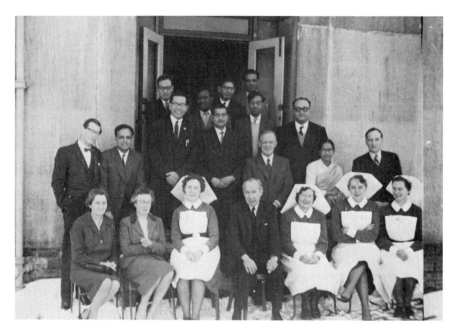

Fig. 31   Dr Alastair Wright is in the centre of a group of staff and postgraduate students (from all over the world) posing for this photograph in the snow in February 1962. Dr Bill Conacher is standing on the left of the second row, and Dr Joyce Grainger is second from the left in the front row.

An invitation to tea with Miss Campbell was a delightful experience. She had a fascinating sitting room next to Ward 9 where she offered true Highland hospitality typical of the little village of Plockton from which she came. There was also a big fire blazing in the hearth with two large armchairs on either side and a large china cabinet crammed full of all her treasures, but the main feature of the room was an enormous dining room table, laden with sandwiches and home baking.

It was in 1951 that I first met Janet Worling who was to become and remain a very close friend. We had both heard of each other but never met until she greeted me at lunch on her first day at Bangour. At that time she was resident house officer in the obstetric and gynaecology unit. She became a living legend as far as the women of West Lothian were concerned. They had complete faith in her and deservedly so. She was a superb practical obstetrician and a gynae-cologist with an uncommon degree of common sense and under-standing of her patients' anxieties, as another colleague wrote in her obituary, and I never had any hesitation in referring patients or colleagues' wives to her.

In May 1955 she was appointed senior registrar which, with Anne Sutherland in the plastic surgery unit and myself, meant that there were three women senior registrars in the hospital. This was quite a change from 1949 when I had first been appointed. A male colleague at that time was heard to comment on my appointment that he wondered how he would ever manage working with a female registrar.

Apart from short spells at the Simpson and Elsie Inglis hospitals in Edinburgh, Janet Worling devoted her whole professional career to Bangour and the women of West Lothian. She was responsible for the development of Bangour's Obstetric Department and very deservedly became its consultant obstetrician and gynaecologist when this post was created for the first time in 1966.

Six years later Dr Worling found herself and her department the centre of world wide attention with the birth in 1972 of the Bostock quins. It was typical of her that she was most concerned that the babies should be allowed to grow up as part of a normal family and to this end she played down the publicity as much as possible and refrained from even writing about the event in the professional medical journals.

She was, however, always eager to share her knowledge and experience with others and many medical students, student nurses and midwives benefited from her clear incisive instruction based on her own broad experience and her very genuine concern for her patients' well being. Dr Worling married Tom Judge who was later to be appointed consultant geriatrician in Edinburgh. During their early married life they lived in one of the hospital houses which is now part of the laboratory. Her untimely death in 1980 was not only a great personal loss but also a very great loss to the West Lothian community. Her funeral was on Hogmanay and despite icy winds and flurries of snow it was attended by a large number of people from all walks of life in West Lothian, showing more eloquently than any words could express the high regard in which she was held. I will always remember her down to earth common sense combined with compassion and a delightful sense of humour.

During the 1950s and 1960s Bangour was a compact hospital serving its local community. It had its own individual character and was very much a part of West Lothian. Many changes have since taken place especially since the 1970s. A major change at that time was the reorganisation of nursing, when instead of Matrons and Sisters and Home Sisters the nursing profession were all to be graded by numbers. One result of these changes was that some excellent Ward Sisters were promoted away from the clinical scene to administration. About the same time the clinical divisional system was introduced into medical practice and hospital administration. All this led to a change in character of the hospital particularly as it became necessary to increase the staff. The development of Livingston New Town led to many other changes including the Livingston Experiment and the introduction of Hospital Practitioners who spent half their working week in general practice in Livingston and half their working week working in various departments throughout the hospital, according to their individual expertise. One of the first Hospital Practitioners to be appointed was Dr Hamish Barber who subsequently became Professor of General Practice in Glasgow University. Another early appointment was Dr Joe Butt who, as a Hospital Practitioner attached to the medical unit, was instrumental in helping the establishment of a diabetic clinic.

Chapter Six

Nursing Memories

Several members of Bangour's nursing staff devoted their whole careers to the hospital and many still have vivid memories of nursing in the late 1940s and early 1950s. In those days Bangour was without many of the facilities now regarded as essential in running a modern hospital, such as the accident and emergency department and the coronary care unit.

Each ward officially had twenty-eight beds but four more could always be squeezed into the middle of the ward to accommodate emergencies. Each ward took its turn in admitting emergencies for two weeks at a time and these extra beds were invariably filled. Unlike the hospitals in Edinburgh, as a District Hospital serving a community, Bangour had to admit emergency patients every day of every week of the year. Like the Windmill Theatre— it never closed its doors! Somehow, no matter how heavy the demand, Bangour and its nurses always coped.

To begin with there were no night theatre staff; the day staff were always on call, however, and even if called on repeated nights in a row they were still expected to continue with their normal daytime duties. At night the whole of the General Hospital was under the supervision of the Night Superintendent, of whom Winnie Sutherland was one of the most famous. Instead of the 'Lady with the Lamp' she was known as the 'Lady with the Torch' and, no matter what the weather, could be seen making her rounds from ward to ward in the pitch darkness of the Bangour night. One night she was injured in a road accident on the A8, but still managed to walk all the way up the Farm Road to be on time for duty in her ward before consenting to be examined when it was discovered that she had a fractured pelvis. Winnie allowed herself only one concession: when the other members of staff all had to go to the staff dining room if they wished anything to eat or drink during the long night shift, she demanded and always got a pot of tea served in her office at exactly 3 a.m.

All ward sisters were a force to be reckoned with and each one had her own peculiarities. Nowhere was this better seen than in the surgical wards, wards Q3 and Q4. Although they were directly opposite each other and practised surgery to equally high standards, the regimes which operated within their walls were very different. While Sister Christie in charge of Q4 insisted on everything being immaculate and every bed being exactly in line, her opposite number, Sister Grant, always seemed to abhor tidiness. Nonetheless the same Frankie Grant was renowned for her skills in resuscitation and wound care. Her nurses were always taught that there were three basics in nursing care and these were to ensure that the patients were free of pain, could get adequate sleep and when awake were kept as comfortable as possible. It was everyones ambition to ensure that patients received adequate privacy and were treated, at all times, as human beings. In those days before the accident and emergency department was opened, casualties were often rushed straight into the ward and during the 1950s these included several men injured in a shale mine disaster. All the patients had compound fractures and while many other sisters would have fussed over getting them washed and bathed before they went to theatre, Sister Grant was quite happy that black faces and gray blankets should be the order of the day in Q3 until she was satisfied that her patients were sufficiently better to be bothered with trivialities such as bed baths.

Another ward sister well remembered from this period was Sister Johnston, who was always known as the Parachuting Sister because of her earlier exploits with the army during the war in Egypt.

Not only members of the nursing staff are remembered. One infamous member of the ancilliary staff was the night porter—Mick Kenny. For a start this Irishman was 6′3″ tall, but more than for his stature he is remembered for his adventures, such as the night he lost a body. It was one of Mick's nightly duties to remove bodies from the wards and to take them down to the mortuary using a covered trolley. One bitterly cold winter night with deep snow on the ground, Mick struggled down the hill only to find when he reached the mortuary that the trolley was empty! With the snow still falling fast, Mick retraced his steps but could find no trace of the missing corpse. Accordingly at 1 o'clock in the morning, he turned out all the night duty staff to help in his desperate search. Fortunately the body was found before the Night Superintendent had to be alerted about the incident and big Mick was able to keep his job as night porter for many years to come. Mick is reported to have commented, after the body had been found, 'Now I understand why they are sometimes called stiffs'.

Another night time incident still well remembered by older members of the nursing staff involved one of the local vagrants, who in those days were much more common and used to roam the roads of West Lothian and were periodically admitted to Bangour. This particular gentleman of the road had enjoyed one too many drinks and no sooner had he been admitted than he vanished. All the nurses were turned out to search for him but no trace could be found of the missing patient and as morning dawned they confessed what had happened to the ward sister, dreading what she would say. They were much relieved when she declared, 'Well, I hope you locked the door after him'. Just at that moment the gentleman in question returned of his own volition. 'What do you mean by giving my nurses all this trouble?' demanded sister. 'You are much too late for breakfast, but I am prepared to give you two tablespoonfuls of epsom salts in hot water!'

A large general and psychiatric hospital like the Bangour complex is rather like a jig-saw puzzle, made up of many different pieces without any one of which it would not be complete. Into this category comes the West Lothian College of Nursing and Midwifery.

The first official recognition of nursing education at the Bangour Hospitals came in 1925 when the General Nursing Council for Scotland approved a school at Bangour Village Hospital for the training of nurses on the mental part of its register. It is known however, that a school had existed before then in the Village Hospital but no approval or inspection of its courses or methods of training were sought.

The training of nurses for work both in Bangour and other Scottish mental hospitals continued within the Village until 1939, when the evacuation of the patients at the start of the war led to the General Nursing Council for Scotland temporarily suspending its recognition of training for the duration of the hostilities.

The creation of Bangour General Hospital during the war, led in the post war years to the need for general nursing training and the General Nursing School was finally officially established in 1950 with Miss Loudon as Tutor in Sole Charge. In the first intake of students were several registered mental nurses from Bangour Village Hospital, who were seconded to complete a second training in general nursing. Among the nursing staff still working at Bangour at the time of the move to St John's Hospital at Howden in 1989, there are several who were among the first students at the new General Nursing Training School in the early 1950s. They include Mrs Mary Ousby the Assistant Director of Nursing Services responsible for the obstetric and gynaecology department, Sister Sanderson in charge of the accident and emergency department, Mr Joe Brown in E.N.T. theatres, Miss Rose Matchett the Night Superintendent, Sally Harkins in charge of the medical out patient department and many more besides. All have vivid memories of their introduction to nursing, which was very much a baptism of fire.

The whole three years and three months of the general nursing course was strictly residential and looking back the former Bangour students felt that embarking on the course was like setting off for a boarding school, as one group of nurses explained:

Weeks before we were due to start we each received a long and very detailed list of uniform, right down to the required liberty bodice. As soon as we arrived we discovered that by uniform they meant uniform.

We had to be immaculate or face the wrath of the sister tutor and it remained that way right through our course as can be seen from our graduation photograph when not one skirt length varied so much as a fraction of an inch above ground level, irrespective of the height of the graduate.

Uniform was the immediate visible sign of the discipline which Bangour Nursing College demanded. The sisters were all ex-army or navy and brought their standards of military discipline with them. It was easier for the smaller number of male nursing students. The men had all been in the forces and had previous experience of this kind of rigid authority and knew how the rules could occasionally be bent. There were four yearly intakes each of fifteen students and it was not uncommon for as many as half of the students to drop out. On the very first day it was made absolutely clear that the first 12 week preliminary training period was strictly probationary and anyone who did not come up to the standard would be asked to leave.

For those who survived, each new day began with prayers, which were compulsory. Then came breakfast in the dining room, where the students of each year sat at long separate tables. Any student who dared to arrive so much as a second after the grace had been said had to make a public apology to Sister Docherty who was in charge of the nurses' home. It was a well known fact that Sister Docherty hated all nursing students, reserving all her love and affection for her cats— two Persian beauties. We saw these two carefully groomed creatures anytime we dared knock on the door of her office. There they sat on an easy chair purring away as we plucked up courage to ask for such a thing as a new tin of the strictly rationed Thomson Cleaner. 'What have you done with the last one?' demanded Sister Docherty. 'Don't you know there is such a thing as elbow grease?'

If getting a tin of cleaner out of Sister Docherty was difficult, obtaining a late pass was impossible. According to the rules of the Bangour Nursing College they could be issued to students on the occasion of special events, but according to Sister Docherty there were no late passes and her word was law. Nor were there any male visitors. Not even husbands were allowed within the hallowed precincts of the nurses' home.

In the end we decided to get our own back and planned a spot of

facing page Fig. 32   The Diploma awarded to nurses after completing their three years training. Catherine Sanderson, 'Sandy', who started her training in 1955, continues to look after the people of West Lothian. Now Senior Sister in the Accident and Emergency Department in the St John's Hospital at Howden. Sister Sanderson was awarded the MBE in the Queen's Birthday Honours List in 1991.

West Lothian (Bangour) Hospital Group Board of Management

Bangour General Hospital

Broxburn

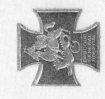

This Certificate is awarded to

Catherine Sanderson

who has been trained at this Hospital in General Nursing for a period of

Three years, passed the Hospital Examinations, and the Final

Examination of the General Nursing Council for Scotland.

Janet R. Lang

Chairman of Nursing Committee

~~Medical Superintendent~~

M Bradley

Matron

Date 11·1·58·

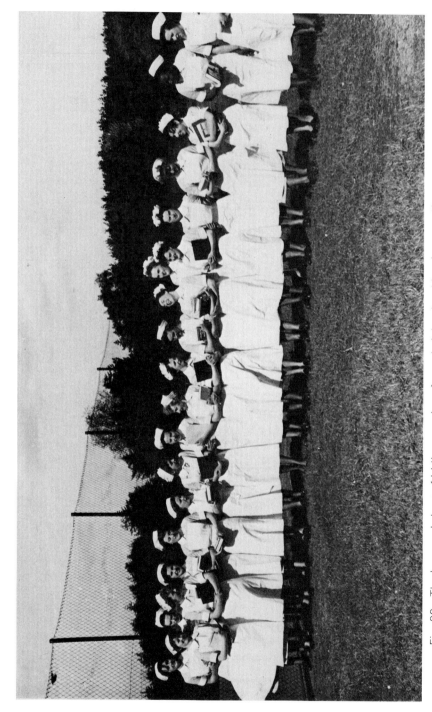

Fig. 33 The long and short of it! 'Irrespective of your height, the skirt of your uniform had to be exactly 14 inches above the ground', recalls one of the former student nurses.

catnapping. Somehow or another the two fluffy Persians were enticed out of the comfort of Sister Docherty's office and despatched in the bottom of one of the big wicker hampers bound for the laundry. Fortunately for them, and probably for us, their mewing was heard before they ended up in the tub along with the dirty sheets.

Meanwhile our studies progressed. The preliminary training period was packed with elementary anatomy and physiology, health and nutrition, theory and practice of cookery, first aid, principles and practice of nursing, history of nursing and social aspects. Visits were arranged to a health clinic, the hospital dairy, the Bangour water works and even the sewage plant. Then, at last, at the start of the seventh week we were actually allowed to spend three hours on observation in a ward.

According to the Bangour Nursing College Prospectus—'The student so gets a grounding in the basic subjects, including the terminology and practice of Elementary Nursing, before she actually works in the ward. During the last six weeks of the twelve week preliminary training period, the student visits the wards for three hours weekly, so that she is introduced gradually into the ward atmosphere.'

The use of the word 'she' throughout was not accidental. Sex discrimination acts had never been heard of in the 1950s and the few male nursing students were viewed with deep suspicion by the sisters. They were not even allowed to appear in the final graduation photograph and were not allowed full recognition by the General Nursing Council.

But before long we had to face the first exams. Preliminary State Examinations had to be taken at the end of the first six months, and the week before we were allowed to revise. That was our first winter at Bangour and, like so many others, was bitterly cold and we either sat huddled in a blanket in our tiny bedrooms in the nurses' home or congregated in the equally spartan and freezing sitting room, where we used up spoonfuls of our tiny rations of sugar, which we each kept in our own little tins, by sprinkling them on the coals of the open fire in an effort to coax it into glowing life.

We passed the exams and from then on the course became much more practical with us working shifts on the wards. It remained as cold as ever with the wind whistling through the long corridors linking the wards, with two feet of snow on the ground outside and totally inadequate heating indoors. The TB patients often joked that they were warmer sleeping out on the verandahs with their covers and their hot water bottles than they would be sleeping in the wards.

The day shift began at 7.30 a.m., relieving the night duty staff who had been on duty since 8 o'clock the previous evening. The big event of the morning was Matron's rounds. Matron Wilson always arrived in the black official car, chauffeur driven by Johnny Cole in his black uniform complete with peaked cap and so it was not surprising that

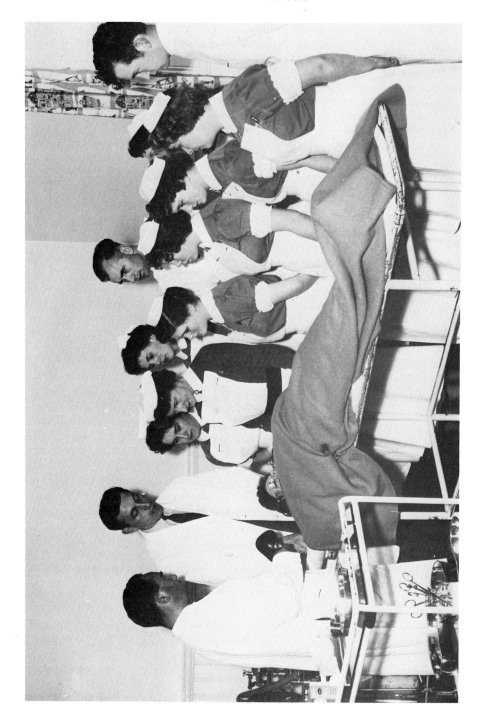

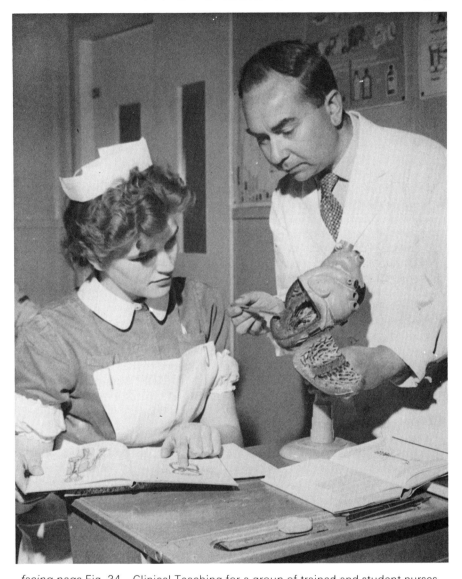

facing page Fig. 34   Clinical Teaching for a group of trained and student nurses.

above Fig. 35   A student nurse is fascinated by the structure and function of the heart.

she became nicknamed 'The Black Widow'. Before her arrival we had to polish and polish the ward floor with heavy wooden bumpers, but we still quaked in terror in case she should find so much as a single speck of dust. She even inspected the wheels of the beds to make sure that they were all exactly in line. We even joked that she expected the patients to turn over strictly in line.

To us, the different sisters we encountered on each ward to which we were allocated as students were every bit as terrifying as the Matron. Sister Chisholm from the Western Isles used to demand of each student, 'And where do you come from?' If you were able to reply 'The Highlands' in the correct accent you were all right and were allocated the treatment room to clean out, otherwise you were sent to slop out the sluice room.

Three months of each of our three years as students were spent on night duty, which meant twelve hours without even a sitting room to take a break. Looking back those long night shifts had their funny moments, but we did not always appreciate them at the time, such as the arrival of the Night Superintendent, Sister Winnie Sutherland. She always seemed able to time her arrival for exactly when we had at last got all the patients settled. Then she would stalk down the ward with her powerful torch. Stopping at a bed at random she would say in her distinct Highland accent, 'Good evening and how are you?' Then, shining the torch straight into the patient's face she would declare, 'Oh, nurse, I see that this patient is still awake.'

At the end of our period of night shift we finished at 8 a.m. and had to start again on day shift at 11 o'clock but at least during the twelve weeks of night shift we enjoyed the luxury of having two whole days off and on both of these mornings we were served breakfast in bed by the maids in the nurses' home.

We had, of course, to pay for the privilege of staying in the nurses' home. It cost so much out of our tiny pay packets that at the end of six months we received the princely sum of £6. This meant that not all of us could afford to travel home, so we used to pool our resources to ensure that we could each go home in turn. For the rest of us the highlight of the week was a walk into Dechmont where we used to buy bottles of lemonade from the little shop in the front room of one of the old cottages.

The lack of diversions did, however, leave us plenty time for study and during the second year block of eight weeks we crammed in the principles of medicine and medical nursing, including communicable diseases, the principles of surgery and surgical nursing, bacteriology, anaesthetics, principles and practice of nursing, social aspects of disease, radiotherapy, physiotherapy and operating theatre techniques!

In the third and final year the teaching block was reduced to six weeks, which made it even more crowded as we were expected to cover, gynaecology and gynaecological nursing, venereal diseases,

diseases of the eye, ear, nose, throat and skin, paediatrics, tuberculosis, burns and ulcers, diets in special diseases, occupational therapy and the social aspects of disease.

At last came the final examinations and at the prize giving which followed we were indeed, as promised in the Bangour Nursing College Brochure, 'presented with the hospital badge and certificate.' Years later that badge with the knight slaying the dragon of disease was the centre of a great controversy, when a landmark was reached in 1969 with the merging of the Bangour Village Hospital Nurse Training School with the General Hospital College, but in the end the badge survived and has been featured in a tapestry which will grace the entrance foyer of the new St John's Hospital at Howden.

In addition to the badges, certificates and prizes, the most distinguished student of each year in both theory and practice received a gold medal, and in our year it was presented to Rose Matchett, who has since gone on to serve Bangour for many years in the operating theatres, accident and emergency department and latterly as Night Superintendent and has become one of the hospital's best known figures.

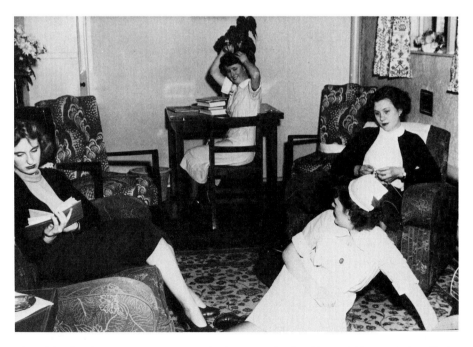

Fig. 36 Student nurses were required to stay in the Nurses' Home during their three years and three months training. In this photograph a group of students are enjoying a few precious moments of unsupervised relaxation; Catherine Sanderson is busy putting up her hair.

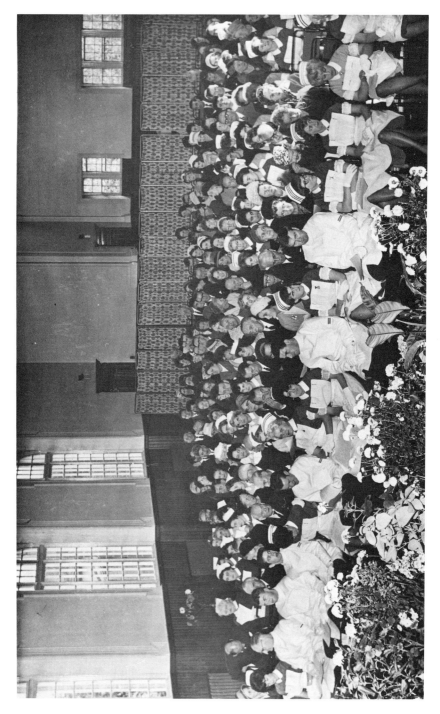

Fig. 37   The Recreation Hall is packed with nurses and their families on Prize Day.

As well as the three year nursing training course, Bangour Nursing College also offered supplementary courses to already qualified nurses such as the Plastic Surgery and Burns Course, the Neuro-Surgical Course and Midwifery Training. For many years during the 1950s the college also provided a special training course for the British Tuberculosis Association Certificate, which was taken by several students who had themselves previously suffered from the disease. In August 1953 the training of midwives for Part II of the Certificate of Midwives Board was begun. The Midwifery Superintendent, Miss E Stewart, as well as being a Registered Midwifery Tutor was also in charge of the clinical midwifery service within the general hospital. In December 1964 the education of midwifery students became a separate entity resulting in the approval and recognition by the Midwives Board of a course leading to State Registration.

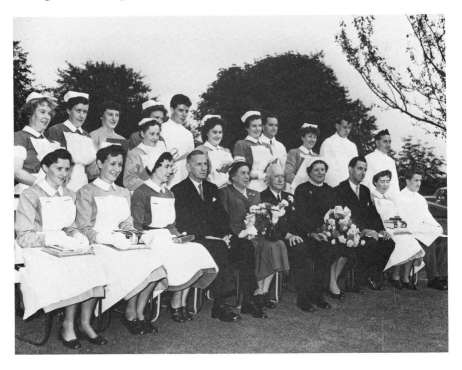

Fig. 38 The Nurses' Prize Day has always been a major occasion in the life of the hospital. Mr Tom Walter Millar, FRCSE (4th left in the front row) then Vice-Chairman of the South East of Scotland Regional Hospital Board, with Miss J D Jolly, Chairman of the General Nursing Council of Scotland (on his left) were presiding at this prize-giving. Mr Millar had previously been the Visiting Consultant Surgeon to the Bangour Hospitals during the war. His son, Dr Geoffrey Millar, is currently on the staff of Bangour and St John's Hospital as a Consultant Opthalmic Surgeon.

The education and training of State Enrolled Nurses commenced in 1959 and was only discontinued in 1986 when it was supplanted by a Bridging Course, enabling selected enrolled nurses to train for the full Nursing Register in either psychiatric or general nursing.

A landmark was reached in 1969 when, as already mentioned, the schools of Bangour Village and General Hospital were amalgamated to form the Bangour Group School of Nursing. Here, training for the Mental and General Registers came together under the same roof at the General Hospital. Mr Arthur Hopwood was appointed as Principal Tutor.

In 1974 the status of a 'college' was granted, with the inclusion of the Midwifery School in the West Lothian College of Nursing and Midwifery, under the control of a Director of Nurse Education directly responsible to the Chief Area Nursing Officer of the Lothian Health Board. The training programmes for nurses at Bangour Hospital were soon recognised as being of a high standard and attracted already qualified nurses from all parts of Britain to enhance their qualifications by taking one of Bangour's specialist courses. One of these nurses who later stayed on and still works at Bangour is Sally Harkins. She recalls her arrival in West Lothian and how she knew from the very outset what a special place Bangour occupied in the hearts of the local people.

> Travelling north from London, I had no idea how far out of Edinburgh Bangour Hospital was situated, so, on arrival at Waverley, I summoned a taxi. As we drove on and on into the darkness beyond the city I realised that the fare was going to be a lot more than I had in my purse. 'How much will that be?' I gulped, when at last we finally pulled up outside the nurses' home.
>
> 'Forget it dear,' replied the driver, 'I owe Bangour a lot more than a taxi fare,' and he then drove off into the night.

Chapter Seven

Accident and Emergency Services
The Killer A8

In December 1969 Mrs J D Kidd, the wife of Lieutenant Colonel Kidd, OBE, chairman of the West Lothian Hospitals Board of Management, opened the new Accident and Emergency Department and Surgical Out Patient Consultation Unit at Bangour General Hospital. These departments had previously been shared in ward Q2 of the surgical block, but they had now been separated and upgraded, together with an extension of the X-Ray Department, at a cost of £126,000. The South East of Scotland Regional Health Board had agreed to this hospital building programme for West Lothian because of the number of road traffic and industrial accidents in the area.

In developing the accident and emergency services, particular attention had been paid to the provision of spacious facilities for the resuscitation and X-Ray investigation of seriously injured patients as well as providing good accommodation for the examination of seriously ill surgical and medical cases.

In an article in the *Lothian Courier* dated 26 December 1969 (not a public holiday in those days) it was reported that, 'Already this year the hospital has dealt with 545 road traffic accidents out of which 187 people have had to be admitted. In 1965 the accident and emergency department had 4,533 new patients. By the end of this year this figure will have risen to 7,400— an increase of 60 per cent in four years'.

Before the completion of the M8 motorway linking Glasgow and Edinburgh in September 1970, the A8 (now the A89) was the main road running across the central belt of Scotland, connecting Edinburgh and Glasgow and passing through the industrial heartland of Scotland. As a result this three-lane highway carried a heavy volume of traffic. This road acquired its unenviable reputation as the 'killer A8' during the 1950s and 1960s when numerous road traffic accidents occurred, involving many serious injuries and deaths. Much of the universal recognition Bangour General Hospital enjoyed throughout the medical world can be directly attributed to the excellence of the surgical services which developed as a result of the vast amount of casualties coming into the hospital from accidents occurring on the A8.

There were notorious 'black spots' along the West Lothian stretch of the A8. Among the worst must be listed the Kilpunt Junction in Broxburn; Pumpherston Crossroads (without traffic lights until October 1968); Dechmont Junction; Livingston Station Road End (now Deans roundabout); Starlaw Junction and Boghead Crossroads at Bathgate; Whitdale Crossroads; and, furthest to the west, Polkemmet Junction. Three main problems can be identified as contributing to this high accident rate when looking at the construction of the A8. First of all, as indicated above, the subsidiary roads running north to south in West Lothian resulted in a high number of crossroads and junctions; secondly, the A8 was at this time a three-lane highway with a shared central overtaking lane; thirdly, nearly all of these junctions were without the benefit of overhead lighting to help visibility during the hours of darkness. It must also be remembered that in the 1950s and 1960s, car headlights were very inferior to modern car lighting systems.

Unfortunately it has not been possible to find a detailed breakdown of the timing of road traffic accidents and the types of vehicles principally involved from the 1950s and 1960s. There is no evidence to suggest that the majority of accidents occurred during the hours of darkness, but traffic density would be reduced at night, therefore there would be the inevitable tendency for people to drive faster. The principal factors in the construction of the A8 giving rise to its high death toll would appear to be the number of crossroads and the shared central overtaking lane. Following the report of an accident which occurred a short distance west of Bangour Farm entrance, the editorial of the *Lothian Courier* dated 2 Feburary 1968 read:

> Drivers fear the A8 generally and this stretch in particular. Some blame restricted vision because of the brow of the hill; the hill is not steep but is deceiving especially to drivers of small or low slung cars.
>
> Another hazard is that traffic to Bangour General Hospital from the east using the Farm Road has to cut into the centre lane of the A8 and wait before crossing into the side road.

Access both to Bangour Village Hospital and Bangour General Hospital when travelling west remains a hazardous experience even in 1990 because drivers of vehicles turning right on the present A89 must take their lives in their hands while waiting for a break in the traffic flow to allow them to enter the hospital.

It might be possible to challenge the conclusion that flaws in the construction of the A8 were responsible for many of the accidents which occurred on this road. While authorities on modern road building techniques accept that the design of a safe road is an important factor in reducing accident rates, much responsibility must remain with the people using the road. One fact which cannot be questioned is that accident rates on the A8 were very high. This can be illustrated by combining some fairly simple accident reports covering a number of years with a detailed list of accidents which took place over one five month period in 1968. In the four years between June 1963 and June 1967 there were 372 accidents on the West Lothian stretch of the A8. Casualties from the accidents totalled 759 of whom 73 died, an average of 18 deaths a year over a 10 mile stretch of road.

An individual look at each of the accidents reported between the beginning of January and the end of May 1968 reveals that this rate showed alarming signs of accelerating. The first accident of the new year occurred on 13 January when a man was killed after a three vehicle crash near the Middleton Hall roadend. Less than a week later, on 18 January, nine people were taken to Bangour after a heavy lorry crashed into the back of a double decker bus which had stopped to allow a woman to alight. This accident occurred only a few hundred yards west of the hospital entrance. The alighting passenger was thrown to the ground, sustaining serious leg injuries, as the stairway from the upper deck of the bus caved in. Firemen, as well as ambulance men, were required on this occasion and hydraulic cutting equipment was used on the buckled stairway to free passengers imprisoned on the top deck.

On the same evening and, again, close to Bangour General Hospital a man sustained fatal injuries when his car collided with another during heavy traffic. The young man killed on this occasion was 23-year-old Joe Serafini from Bathgate, a talented golfer who was known throughout Scotland. Joe had won a Scottish Universities cap during his final year at Strathclyde and great things had been expected from him in the sport of golf.

Before January was over another Bathgate man was killed outright and his passenger seriously injured in a three-vehicle accident early in the morning of the 31st. The crash occurred at almost precisely the same spot as those which had taken place only two weeks previously.

Three accidents within a fortnight and three deaths within a month prompted the *Lothian Courier* of 2 February to ask, 'Is there a hoodoo on this stretch of the A8?'

Indeed February showed little sign of improvement when three accidents occurred, this time not within a fortnight but within seven hours of each other, on Wednesday, 7 February. Amazingly no one was killed, but a child of seven sustained severe head injuries and was transferred in a critical state to the Edinburgh Royal Infirmary, and a motorist from Fife was taken to Bangour General Hospital's Plastic Surgery Unit.

March and April passed by uneventfully but May saw the 'killer' road strike again, increasing its toll of fatalities for the year. On 27 May three local young men were killed in an accident involving a mini and a lorry at the

Starlaw Road Junction, Bathgate. The accident occurred in thick fog. Three days later, on 30 May, one man died and three others were injured in an early morning collision on the stretch between Little Boghead, Bathgate and Whitdale near Whitburn.

Even from this basic survey of a relatively short period of time the dangers of the A8 are apparent. In the five months studied there were seven separate major accidents almost all of which involved the loss of life. Three of these accidents occurred at almost exactly the same spot, very close to the Bangour Hospitals, and although it has already been suggested that the entrance to the hospital may well have been a factor in causing these accidents, the point must also be made that more lives might well have been lost had it not been for the close proximity of the hospital and the excellent service provided by its staff.

One patient, Robert Gibson of Livingston Station, then aged 21, was admitted on 12 June 1965 in a serious condition following a road accident. Mr Gibson was unconscious on admission with extensive scalp and facial lacerations and depressed fractures of the middle third of his face. In addition he had a shattered fracture of the proximal third of his right femur (thigh bone), a fracture of his right knee cap and severely displaced fractures of both bones of the right forearm. Detailed and extensive surgery was undertaken by Mr Alastair Bachelor and Mr Noel Gray. Mr Gibson was subsequently able, as the hospital discharge letter notes, to go home on 31 August 1965, 'walking without crutches, all wounds having healed satisfactorily'.

In the same accident, on 12 June 1965, William Wilson, also aged 21, of Bathgate was admitted. His main injuries consisted of severe intra abdominal bleeding requiring immediate laparotomy; a compound shattered fracture of his right femur (thigh bone); transverse fracture of the left humerus (arm bone); compound fracture of the right elbow with displacement of the olecranon; bilateral fractures of the pelvic bone, and bilateral collapsed lungs requiring immediate drainage. Mr Wilson was unconscious on admission and remained semi-conscious for several days. After recovering from extensive surgery following his accident, and overcoming the life threatening complication of long bone fracture known as a fat embolus which developed, Mr Wilson was able to walk out of hospital with only minimal assistance from crutches on 30 August 1965. In a letter to Mr Wilson's employers on 2 August 1965 written by the late Mr John G Clark, FRCS, who was Surgical Registrar at Bangour Hospital at that time, Mr Wilson was said to be continuing to make an excellent recovery and that he had every prospect of being able to return to his former employment with the Post Office. Mr John G Clark tragically died in 1969 of serum hepatitis which he contacted as a result of his pioneering work in renal transplant surgery in the Edinburgh Royal Infirmary.

The third seriously injured victim of this dreadful accident was Sarah

Wilson. Sarah also required an emergency abdominal operation. Sarah had been admitted to hospital for observation of what were initially thought to be relatively minor injuries following the accident. She collapsed while in the ward in 'shock' due to blood loss and an exploratory abdominal operation was undertaken to identify the cause. At surgery Sarah was found to have ruptured her womb and to have bled extensively into the abdominal cavity. Tragically Sarah was 5 months pregnant and she lost her baby but it was possible to repair the womb. Thereafter Sarah made an excellent recovery, with the help of a blood transfusion of 5 pints, and she was able to go home on 23 June 1965. This part of the story has a happy ending because Sarah eventually married and subsequently bore two children.

The fourth victim of the accident was Barbara Wilson, William Wilson's sister. Fortunately her injuries of concussion, extensive bruising and minor lacerations around the face did not require surgery and she was able to go home on 16 June 1965.

Not every one was as lucky as the Gibsons and Wilsons, being able to go home within a few weeks of their various accidents. District Councillor Jimmy McGinley, Representative for Linlithgow's Preston Ward gained a vivid patient's eye view of Bangour General Hospital when, as a young man, he was seriously injured in a motor cycle accident and spent many months in ward Q3.

I spent my twenty-first birthday in ward Q3 at Bangour. I can't remember all that much about it but I can recall the staff around my bed and the candles all lit! I thought, well, if this is heaven, then death is nothing to worry about. Mind you in a busy emergency ward, they had enough to do especially as I had been admitted only one week earlier with serious multiple injuries as the result of an accident. I have never forgotten that team of doctors and nurses.

As a Bathgate Bairn, Bangour had been my local hospital. Staff were recruited from all over but naturally a large number of them were recruited locally—girls that I went to school with, I knew them and I knew their families. Many of the staff came from my own home town or were courting or married to boys from my home town. The unique point was that I always had to address them as Staff Nurse ... or Nurse ...—never, never, Mary or Judith. The Ward Sister would have disciplined the girls severely if the patients had shown any familiarity. The Ward Sister, in those days, was a 'holy terror' to the staff but to the patients she was a woman in a million. I may have been 21-years-old but, by heavens, she could put me in my place if I stepped over the mark. Not that I could really, because I was bed bound with a Thomas Splint on my shattered leg from May to November. I can assure you it is no picnic being suspended on a system of pulleys and weights from a beam over the bed, with only your head, shoulders and one leg resting on the bed.

Anyhow, after a few weeks, it was decided that I could be put on occupational therapy to get my arm and fingers working again. By the time the next four months had elapsed the staff were nearly climbing the walls. My mate and I recruited all the ten to fourteen short stay and day patients who were in for minor surgery. We used them to do the rough work on our handicrafts and we finished them off. The list included:

> trays, baskets of all shapes and sizes, soft toys of all shapes and sizes, toys like pandas (extremely popular in the 1950s). The pandas we made ranged from 3 inches high to 2 feet high. Purses, wallets, writing cases, engraved work.

Orders came from staff and employees all over the hospital, visitors and friends too. To this day I still have two of my pandas, Mickey Mouse, rabbits and Leo the Lion. Later, as an out patient, the pace continued in the workshop and today I still use the coffee tables I made. That period in my life was most certainly an unforgettable experience and I came out of hospital with £407 in the bank as a

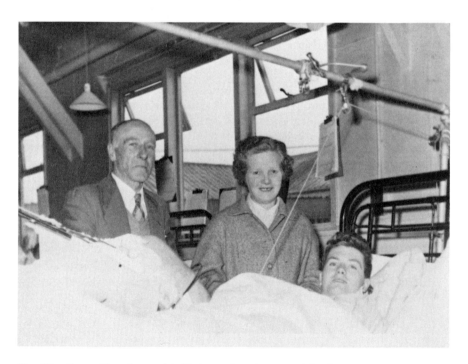

Fig. 39 Councillor Jimmy McGinley enjoyed many visits from his parents during his long stay in Ward Q3 following his motor-bike accident on his twenty-first birthday. Here he is seen flat on his back with a Balkan Beam and Thomas Splint to treat his broken thigh.

result of the toys that I had made. Mind you it gives an idea of the amount of work we put in when you realise that we charged 5 shillings for a purse, seven and sixpence for a wallet and the toys ranged from 10 shillings to £1 each.

In addition, to help pass the time, we used to play all manner of card games, dominoes, draughts and chess. I had never really done any of these things before so it can be said that I used my time in hospital to improve my social graces.

Like everyone else, whether in hospital or not, you have your good days and your bad days. Bribing the staff to leave the T.V. on late in those days was 'mission impossible'—but we used to try! 'Nurse, nurse,' I would call. 'Yes James, what is it?' 'Can we see the film at 10.15 p.m.?' Answer: No. 'Please, I won't ask for a bed pan on your shift if you let us watch the T.V.' 'Oh, I see, well what if Night Sister or Matron come on their rounds unexpectedly—do you think you can jump out of that bed to switch it off!' 'Sorry—No.'

Sometimes we were successful and had some great ideas that would make prison camp movie makers jealous of the plots. However I am not going to tell you these stories because we patients do have our code of ethics, but, sometimes we did manage to watch the T.V.

After I had left hospital, I remember one day when I wasn't long married walking down Leith Walk in Edinburgh with my newly wed wife towards Valvona & Crolla, the delicatessen shop. A tall man was putting items in the boot of his car. I said to my wife—'I know that man, that's Mr. Gray, the Surgeon who operated on me. I think I will go over and say hello and ask him how he thinks I am managing, two years after my accident.'

I took my courage in both hands. 'Hello sir, how are you?' I said. He looked at me and immediately smiled and said, 'You're the young man with the compound fractured femur, compound fractured tibia and fibula and the fractured pelvis—what was your name again?' I was quite amazed—after all what's in a name.

One particular double fatal accident which occurred in 1964 is worthy of mention because of the ensuing mess. The accident took place on the A8 near to Livingston Station Road End when a private motor car was in collision with a lorry conveying about 10 tons of bulk Apricot Jam, which spilt out onto the road. Recalling the accident Superintendent Donald Mackinnon, at that time an enquiry officer, describes how 'all the services were wading in a pool of jam which was 2 feet deep in places.' In the process of cleaning it up all the drains in the area were blocked and the corridors of the Accident and Emergency Department at Bangour General Hospital were 'as treacherous as an ice rink'.

As fear of the killer road grew throughout the 1950s and 1960s, so did pressure for improvements to the A8. Two such improvements materialised

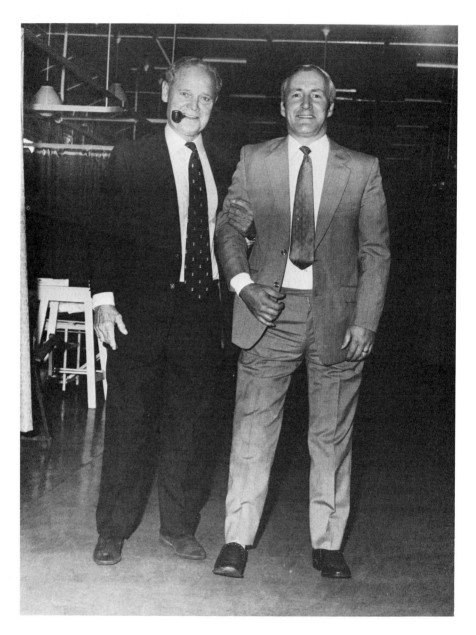

Fig. 40 Two men, no legs, bags of courage. 'Reach for the Sky' Second World War fighter pilot Douglas Bader (left), who lost both legs in a plane crash, found time to visit the physiotherapy department at Bangour to encourage Jimmy Dunne during his rehabilitation after a serious accident.

in 1968 but even then they were not given a universal welcome. In June that year the new pedestrian overbridge on the A8, opposite the entrance to Bangour Village Hospital was opened but at a meeting of the West Lothian Roads Committee it was criticised as being 'hopeless' for the elderly and for people attending the hospital. This criticism came from Councillor Miss Jean Paris who claimed that the thirty-two steps were far too steep. Mr James McCance, County Road Surveyor, explained that the bridge was built by the Scottish Development Department and was of traditional design. He added, oddly enough since it still stands in 1991, that the bridge would be removed when the new M8 motorway was completed. Presumably it was either to be replaced with another bridge or the Scottish Development Department felt that, once the M8 was in operation, the A8 might be crossed safely by pedestrians without needing to use the bridge. The other significant improvement of the year took place in October when high speed traffic signals, the first of their kind in Scotland, were installed at the Pumpherston Crossroads. The idea of these new lights was that they were operated by a 'magic eye' which would allow fast moving traffic to pass through the lights before they changed. They were thus designed specifically to avoid the necessity of sudden braking when approaching the junction, thereby, it was hoped, reducing the risk of accident. Their installation was again paid for by the Scottish Development Department and although the lights were greeted with some scepticism at first, they were generally seen as a step in the right direction.

Important as these improvements were, the huge and overriding desire among the residents of West Lothian and users of the A8 was to see the new M8 in operation as soon as possible! The universal hope was that, once opened, the new motorway would draw the teeth of the killer A8. Although construction of the M8 was almost complete by the late 1960s, the West Lothian stretch was the last to be built and work on the 7 miles between Whitburn and Dechmont did not begin until early 1968. The building of the M8 brought problems of its own to the A8, especially when the final stretch between Dechmont and Newbridge got underway in 1969. When this work began, it involved closing the section of the A8 running from Bangour Hospital to the Dechmont roundabout and diverting all A8 traffic through the village of Dechmont. As the speed limit on the West Lothian stretch of the A8 at the time was 50 mph, the diversion was not seen as immensely dangerous. This opinion was immediately revised however when it was announced that the speed limit was to be raised to 70 mph from early 1970. The following extract from the *Lothian Courier* dated 26 February 1969 relates the controversy surrounding the announcement.

The speed limit on the A8 is to be raised from 50 to 70 mph as from January 5th 1970. The news, contained in a letter from Mr. Keeley of the Scottish Home Department to Mr. J. Little, secretary of Dechmont Community Association, fills the villagers with dread. Traffic will be coming towards the village at high speed before motorists realise what is happening and can reduce to 30 mph.

Mr. Little, in writing to Mr. Tam Dalyell, M.P. for West Lothian, to thank him for his past help in the matter of the Dechmont traffic, adds in respect of Mr. Keeley's letter: 'This is madness. How do they hope to keep death off the roads? What possible chance would school children have? How can a motorist be expected to suddenly slow down from 70 to 30 mph?'

At a later point in this article the *Lothian Courier* goes on to report that a spokesman for the Scottish Information Office had confirmed that the speed limit on the whole of the A8, with the exception of those sections travelling through villages, would be raised to 70 mph.

Originally [said the spokesman], when the 3 lane A8 was carrying all traffic between Edinburgh and Glasgow, it was felt wise to impose a 50 mph limit on stretches such as that in front of Bangour Village Hospital. However, now that the motorway is in operation from Dechmont westwards and a pedestrian bridge has been provided in front of the hospital, it is felt that there is really no longer any need for the 50 mph speed limit and, from January 5th, the limit on the A8 will be 70 mph, the limit which applies in general.

Although the immediate fears of the Dechmont residents in fact proved to be unfounded, it was with much relief that the final section of the M8 was opened in September 1970. The objective of 37 miles of motorway between the boundaries of Edinburgh and Glasgow was finally achieved and the black years of the killer A8 were over. With the opening of the M8, the A8 was no longer required to serve two incompatible purposes, namely, as the main road carrying all Edinburgh/Glasgow traffic, and as the link between various communities in West Lothian, providing all the necessary functions which such communities require—junctions at subsidiary roads, safe access to a hospital entrance, and access to public transport. It was not just the volume of traffic using the A8 which gave rise to the road's reputation as a killer but the diversity of that traffic. Even today it is still possible to crawl for a good mile or two along the A8 behind a heavy farm vehicle and annoying though this can still be, in the days when the road was carrying all high speed traffic between Glasgow and Edinburgh it was positively dangerous.

As far as Bangour General Hospitsl was concerned the opening of the M8 motorway coincided with the opening of the hospital's new Accident and Emergency Department. It was this unit's predecessor which put the hospital firmly on the map by providing unfailing and invaluable assistance on so many occasions.

In the years 1969 to 1989 it was hoped that the numbers attending the Accident and Emergency Department as a result of road traffic accidents, industrial accidents, accidents in the home and accidents in the pursuit of sport and leisure activities would decline. In this way the department could gradually change from providing an accident service to providing an emergency service for non accident surgical and medical cases. The accompanying table reviews the total number of new patients attending the Accident and Emergency Department on an annual basis and indicates the continuing major growth in this area of the hospital's workload, justifying an expansion in the numbers of staff and the appointment of Dr Peter Freeland as Consultant. The department has been involved in many developments including the use of Computer Assisted Diagnosis of abdominal pain, the management of drug overdoses and various other research projects which have been presented at clinical meetings and published in reputable medical journals. The last such publication from the department was undertaken by Dr Fiona McGregor and involved the use of metal staples to close skin lacerations.

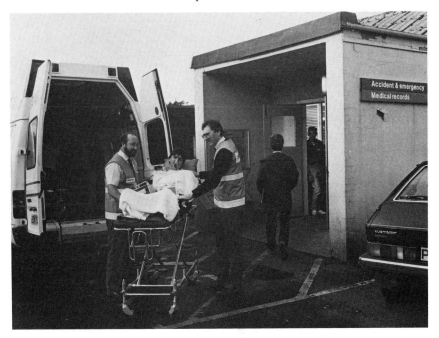

Fig. 41   A typical scene at the front door of Casualty shortly before it closed in 1989.

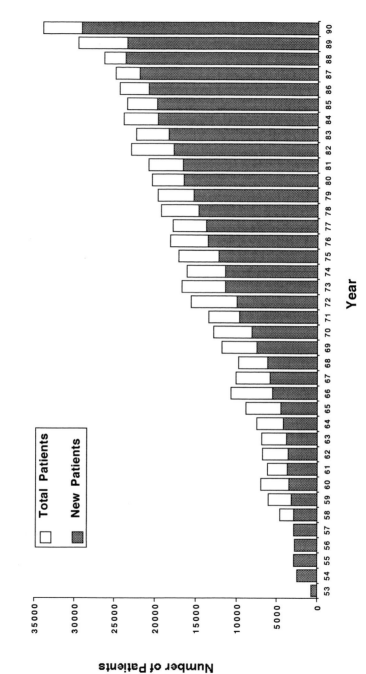

Fig. 42   Graph showing number of patients attending the Accident and Emergency Department of Bangour General Hospital 1953–90.

Chapter Eight

New Faces and New Hope

Mention Bangour anywhere in the country and someone is sure to say, 'Isn't that the famous Burns unit?'

It was the knowledge that a second world war was imminent, and the fear of the heavy casualties and terrible injuries it would produce, that prompted the Government decision of 1939 to establish burns and plastic surgery units in all parts of the country as swiftly as possible. The new Emergency Medical Services Hospital at Bangour Annexe was selected as the best site to serve East and Central Scotland, where the existence of military targets such as the Rosyth Royal Naval Dockyard and the RAF Fighter stations at East Fortune and Turnhouse made the likelihood of heavy casualties in the region almost inevitable.

Many of the original plastic surgery techniques and operations were developed in the early nineteenth century but the growth of the specialty of plastic surgery owed its origins to the badly battle scarred victims of the First World War. During the 1920s and 1930s little advancement had been made in this field of surgery and the specialty had not developed or expanded adequately to provide sufficient experienced staff to serve the new Burns and Plastic Surgery Units being established throughout the country. The Government therefore turned to First World War veteran Sir Harold Gillies to act as its advisor.

Sir Harold used his contacts amongst the medical profession throughout the country to recruit staff whom he realised must be trained quickly for the new specialty of Plastic Surgery. In Edinburgh he approached the then Professor of Surgery, Sir James Learmonth, and asked him to recommend 'a young, up and coming man'. Learmonth's choice was A B Wallace—a name destined to become world famous.

At that time Mr Wallace was busy establishing his reputation in paediatrics at the Royal Hospital for Sick Children in Edinburgh, but he accepted the challenge to set up the new department at Bangour. First he travelled to London, intending to spend six weeks studying under Gillies. His arrival coincided with the start of the blitz, however, and the bombing raids completely disrupted his studies. He returned for a second attempt later and this time he learned much from the acknowledged expert.

By the spring of 1941, building at Bangour was more or less complete and the Burns and Plastic Surgery Department opened in 'T' block. The wards were just as basic as all of the other long huts at Bangour and had little of the highly specialised equipment or air conditioning systems now considered essential for the treatment of severe burns and plastic surgery patients. Even at the time of the closure of Bangour General Hospital none of this equipment has been obtained, but what Bangour always had was dedicated nurses and doctors, all eager to develop their skills.

The staff of the new unit, initially led by Mr A B Wallace, did not have long to wait as all of the sailors badly burnt in the Battle of Narvik were brought to Bangour. Later, in 1942, the Duke of Kent's Sunderland Flying Boat, while setting out on a morale-boosting trip to RAF stations in Iceland, crashed into the 700 feet high Eagle's Rock in Sutherland, probably as a result of a compass error. The sole survivor of the fourteen-man crew, the rear gunner, was rushed south to Bangour. Although he was very badly burned, the expert treatment and nursing he received saved his life and he lived until 1978.

To help with such difficult cases Sir Harold Gillies paid regular three-monthly visits to Bangour. By this time A B Wallace was steadily developing his own skills and went on to gain world-wide recognition when he published his famous 'Rule of Nines' the theory of which was that by dividing the human body into zones each making up 9 per cent of the total body surface, patients' burn injuries could be more accurately assessed and treated.

Mr Wallace also gained great international fame by popularising the exposure method of treating burns. In certain carefully selected cases, he recommended leaving burn injuries without dressings in order to cut down on the risk of infection. This controversial treatment attracted many professional visitors from all over the world to Bangour, but it must be stressed that at no time did Mr Wallace advocate its universal application.

During the war years many of the cases being dealt with at Bangour involved head and facial injuries and Mr Campbell Buchan was summoned from Peel Hospital near Galashiels in the Scottish Borders, where he had been specialising in dentistry, to help manage these complex injuries. Professor Boyd was appointed the first Oral surgeon.

At Bangour the surgeons were backed by a team of technicians and nurses whose skills were constantly improving as they overcame seemingly impossible barriers to the recovery of terribly injured patients. Names which stand out amongst the technicians are those of the highly innovative Stuart Cleary, and Alex Young who started out as Stuart's apprentice and still works at Bangour. No matter how unusual the artificial appliance which the surgeons requested to replace some part of a patient's badly damaged body, the device was painstakingly manufactured by the technicians who took great pride in ensuring that it fitted the patient as precisely as possible.

Although the hours were long and the work demanding the staff also found time for romance. One theatre sister in the unit, Marjory Clark, married Mr Campbell Buchan, while her colleague, Sister Hardy, married a Norwegian serviceman who had been one of her patients.

By 1943 more and more overseas patients were being admitted to the Burns Unit, including some from Norway, Poland and Canada. Nursing them back to health was a long process lasting months, even years. It took a great deal of time for skin grafts to succeed, and if a graft failed to take or became infected the whole slow process had to begin all over again. The loving, caring, dedicated atmosphere of the Burns Unit at Bangour has been vividly described by the author Brenda McBride who, as a young nurse, was sent north from England to learn the techniques which the Scots were pioneering. In her book *A Nurses War* she writes:

> The burns centre at Bangour had come into being as a result of the Battle of Britain in 1940 when so many airmen had been badly burned. After their initial treatment had come the need for plastic surgery, to free joints from binding scar tissue; to build up their new faces again. Here, in Bangour, the work of repair was still going on for some of those Battle of Britain pilots. The unit, built as an emergency hospital, sprawled up a bleak hillside in single-storey, wooden buildings. Pin and I were given a room each in a hut allotted to the civilian staff and were made welcome by the Scottish girls there. That first morning, when we accompanied the surgeons (Mr Wallace and Mr Buchan) and their physiotherapists around the ward was a revelation to us both.
>
> The scarred hands on one RAF pilot were contracted back towards the wrist to a position where they were virtually functionless. His face was young and handsome but his raw, red hands were like a bunch of boiled prawns.
>
> Mr Wallace pointed to the tough cords at the wrist that were immobilising the hands. 'We'll remove all this scar tissue, straighten out the wrist, skin graft the raw area and wrap the whole thing in plaster until it heals. OK?'
>
> The owner of the hands nodded enthusiastically. As I sketched down a diagram in my notebook, it dawned on me that this man was injured in 1940. It was now 1943 and hospital treatment still stretched for months maybe years, ahead of him.
>
> The next patient was sitting with a bundle of cane on his lap and the beginnings of a basket. He was one of the success stories, we were told, but to Pin and me he looked like a major disaster. Three years ago, he had leapt from his burning, spiralling plane, a little knot of flame at the end of a parachute. His limbs were mobile now but his face was still in the process of being rebuilt. The new eyelids were still puffy, still showing the stitchmarks, and the large, round graft on

one cheek was the pale skin of his left buttock that had not yet taken on colour from the face's blood supply. Twin tunnels in a stub of bone was all he had left of a nose. Mindful that our reactions, as newcomers, were being closely observed by these patients, Pin and I were careful to show no emotion.

The surgeon was describing to us the repair he had carried out on the pilot's mouth. 'Contracting muscle was pulling it right over here to the other side of his face and we are very pleased with the correction.'

'That goes for me, too,' said Pilot Officer Humphrey, who still needed lips.

'What we did,' the surgeon went on, 'was to strip a length of fascia from his leg muscle and insert one end here, stitching it to the corner of his mouth. Then we made another incision here by the cheekbone on the same side of the face, inserted long sinus forceps to the corner of the mouth to pick up the free end of the fascia strip, pulled it through and secured it. Now he can smile.'

I tried to nod intelligently and wondered with despair what Mr Humphrey could find to smile about. He was listening intently to everything the surgeon was saying.

'And now we will tackle your nose.' The junior surgeon Mr Buchan took the top off his pen and made a note in his pocket book.

'Great!' said the airman. 'Give me something to blow for Christmas.'

The surgeons bent over Mr Humphrey with a skin marking pencil and sketched a diagram on his forehead. 'There is good skin here and a good hair line. We'll swing down a flap incorporating some hair bearing cells which will be used for nostrils later. The raw area on the forehead will be grafted from the abdomen.'

So it went on, all around the ward, robbing Peter to pay Paul, taking skin from undamaged areas to graft on to denuded places, sometimes planting little islets of skin, leaving them to grow and unite. This was surgery calling for great patience on the part of the surgeon and patient alike, with many trips to the operating theatre before the job was finished.

Then we came to the pedicle grafts, known amongst the men themselves as the 'dangle'ums', which was self explanatory at a certain stage of the repair. Aircraftsman Harding was in the process of receiving a pedicle graft to the badly scarred right side of his face. A tube of flesh had been formed on the calf of one leg by stitching together two sides of an incised rectangle. When the blood supply was established within this tube, one end was freed from the leg and stitched to the palm of the hand. Again, time was allowed for a blood supply to be established between the palm of the hand and the end of the flesh tube, then that end which was still attached to the calf was freed, trimmed to fit and stitched over the burnt area of the face. The patient now had a bridge of flesh between his cheek and his palm and this remained until the cheek itself was seen to be involved in the

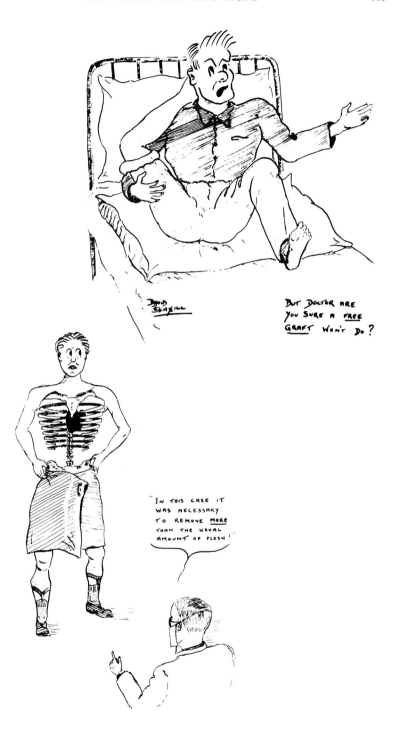

circulation. Then the tube of flesh was removed from the hand and the hand grafted. Now the patient had earned the title of 'Dangle'um' for a pedicle of flesh hung from the cheek, or nose or whatever was being repaired. They made a weird but valiant group, forming themselves into the Dangle'Ums Club with a special membership badge. When the pedicle was seen to have a healthy blood supply from the face, it was trimmed and moulded to make a flesh cheek or nose, a result which could not have been achieved with a thin graft.

Up to now, I'd thought of plastic surgery in connection with face-lifts for aging women. Bangour showed me its real purpose. There were men with burnt elbows stitched inside the raised skin of the abdomen, immobilised there until the graft should 'take'. New lower jaws were fashioned from bottom ribs. Uppers of burnt feet were stitched to the underside of calves. Men with extensive body burns were lowered into warm saline baths and encouraged by physio-therapists to keep muscles flexible with the gentle movements possible under the water. Dressings here did not stick. I remember my burnt children at Newcastle.

Pin and I, in theatre clothing, stood by the operating table while the surgeons sewed gossamer stitches on skin no stronger than the skim on boiled milk, heads bent, working slowly and patiently, sometimes for two hours at a stretch. They encouraged our interest, demonstrating the dermatome, a roller-type instrument for removing skin, and they showed us how the grafts must be dressed. After the initial treatment in the theatre when the grafts were firmly fixed in position with bandages or by plaster of Paris, it was 6 to 10 days before the first dressing was done, depending on the thickness of the skin used. This was a job for either Pin or myself and was always a tense moment. If the graft had 'taken', the patient could move on to the next stage; if not, the operation would have to be repeated at a future date and that would mean more raw donor areas, leaving less skin for grafting.

To remove the last covering and see a dry, healthy graft was as exciting for us as for the patient. If part of the graft had sloughed off and there was pus, then 4 hourly saline packs had to be applied and a swab sent to the pathology department. This was a technique new to us. An infected wound was always investigated for the culprit organism and then treated specifically; elementary one might think, but not standard practice. We filled a notebook with the classification of harmful bacteria and their neutralisers. We learned to remove stitches with delicacy where a shaky hand could undo the miracle worked by the surgeon. We learned the absolute necessity of irrigation after food on stitchlines in the mouth. Minced chicken adhering to a repair of soft palate was no good to anyone. There was a whole new range of instruments for us to memorise, named after their innovators; McIn-doe's fine, tapering dissecting forceps, Gillies' rake retractor, Gillies' needleholder with cutting edge, and many more. This was a new and fascinating field of surgery and the day we removed the plaster from those previously contracted wrists of the pilot was one of the many sublime moments of success. We had seen the operation to free his hands of restricting bands of scar tissue. We had watched while a dermatome graft was applied to the now extended wrists. Now, one week later, it was time to see the result.

There was a bad smell as we cut through the plaster. The airman's nostrils quivered. We removed the cotton wool, the acriflavine gauze and the tulle gras underneath. Slowly, we uncovered a pink, dry graft with only a very small area of subcutaneous haemorrhage. The graft was totally successful and the new, extended position of the wrists was a great improvement. His hands could now be made to work. There was some swelling due to the plaster but the physiotherapist was already dealing with that. It was a moment of acute satisfaction for everyone concerned.

Time passed quickly. Christmas came and was made much of, with free beer, a film show, turkey and pudding. My 'plastic' Christmas was one of the happiest I have ever spent in hospital. Pin was a wonderful nurse. All her natural shyness left her when she was caring for these men. I would look across the ward and see her face lit up as she jollied along some brave buffoon with a paper cap above his own false nose. We kept our pity for when we were alone.

If one were to judge from the general hilarity of the men, it would seem that no one there had a care in the world. One or two went home to their families for the holiday but the majority of these dreadfully mutilated men preferred to stay in hospital and I wondered if the wards, with their freakish inhabitants, had indeed become the real world. New noses, ears and chins were something to boast about here but the outside world could be cruelly inquisitive or too politely ignoring. Out there, they would have to accept sly glances from fellow travellers on the buses, peeps from behind the neighbours' curtains and piercing announcements from small children.

Keeping lively young servicemen occupied during the lengthy periods between their operations was difficult, but the unit was helped greatly by the Canadian occupational therapist Miss de Brisay who taught the men how to weave and how to make seagrass stools. Those who were fit to be up were enlisted to help with the chores around the ward and were also able to avail themselves of the full-sized billiard table in the recreation hall, and the library which was set up by the local Red Cross. For the injured commandos amongst them, however, such pastimes proved far too tame and they put their survival skills training to the test by setting snares so that Bangour's meagre wartime rations were frequently supplemented with rabbit, cooked in every possible way from stew to curry.

A big incentive towards good behaviour amongst the military patients who could walk, was that Ward Sisters had the power to grant passes which, when presented to the Military Registrar who was based at Bangour, meant the luxury of a few hours away from the hospital. For many this simply meant a walk along to Dechmont Village with its post office and shop, but, despite war-time restrictions on public transport, some soldiers managed to enjoy nights out in Bathgate or even Edinburgh. On their return, of course, they always had to be fit to walk all the way up the Farm Road from the main road end of the A8, definitely a sobering experience.

Some entertainment was also provided occasionally at the hospital and this ranged from local concert parties to a celebrated visit by Scotland's top entertainer of the time, Sir Harry Lauder, who was accompanied by his niece Gretta.

All the time, however, the serious work of the Burns Unit continued with operations five days a week. Pressure on the unit reached its height after D Day in 1944 when the number of casualties transported to Bangour was so high that patients were crowded forty to a ward. Dressings were in short supply and sphagnum moss in gauze bags, a technique which had been used successfully in the First World War, was again pressed into service because of its absorbent and antiseptic properties. So many operations were performed that reserves of blood began to run low and a local appeal for help brought a tremendous response from the people of West Lothian.

At the same time that the hospital was coping with this large increase in acute patients, word was received that two wards had immediately to be made available to house male and female geriatric patients, who were being evacuated from London because their beds were needed for the casualties of Hitler's dreaded 'Doodlebug' flying bombs.

Throughout all this activity the Matron of the Bangour Hospitals, Miss McNaughton, was insistent that nothing must in any way disrupt the smooth running of the Plastic Surgery and Burns Unit, whose number of admissions reached its peak in 1945. Later that year the end of the war in the Far East brought home a flood of servicemen, many of whom needed extensive reconstructive surgery to rebuild their shattered faces.

Peacetime did not bring an end to such terrible cases and the steady increase in road traffic brought many crash casualties, especially among motor cyclists; these ranged from skilled riders, such as army despatch riders, to young men who had wrecked their first bikes. Sadly motor cyclists continue to feature in the department's statistics, and to a far greater extent than their numbers would justify when compared with those of other road users.

Prior to government legislation making it compulsory for anyone travelling in the front of a car to use seatbelts, the plastic surgeons spent many months rebuilding the faces, where possible, of the victims of head-on car crashes who had hit the shattered windscreen, dashboard or steering wheel.

Trying to prevent the tragedy of avoidable road traffic, industrial or domestic accidents and burns has ensured that many staff have taken a leading role in Accident Prevention Organisations such as ROSPA (Royal Society for the Prevention of Accidents), MCAP (Medical Commission on Accident Prevention) and SAPC (Scottish Accident Prevention Council). Mr A C H Watson, Consultant Surgeon in the Plastic Surgery Unit, has worked tirelessly for many years to prevent burning and scalding accidents in children.

Industrial injuries also provided a steady flow of patients, including one of Bangour's longest attending patients, Mrs Jessie Jardine, who was injured in a munitions explosion in Dumfries.

One of the main difficulties in saving the lives of patients in the Burns Unit used to be ensuring that they got sufficient nourishment. Two of Bangour's staff, Anne Sutherland, who was originally a dietician, and Alastair Batchelor, who was at the time a senior registrar, contributed greatly to this area of research by conducting a large scale project into the feeding of serious burn victims.

Alastair Batchelor, who later became the Senior Consultant Surgeon within the unit, recalls the close-knit nature of the department and the friendly, almost family atmosphere of the Burns Unit.

> On the patients' side this was partly because so many of them stayed in the wards for much longer than most patients have to do nowadays. On the medical side this closeness resulted from so many of us staying in the residency or, at most, no further away than Dechmont village. We were also supported by good colleagues in other departments such as Dr Robert Saffley, the radiologist, who was one of the gentlemen of this world.
>
> The administration of the hospital ran like clockwork under Mr Robert Ross and his very able secretary, Miss Paton. The Hospital Board met regularly once a month under the well known Chairman of Scottish Oils, Mr Robert Crichton who was very much a father figure to the hospital. All the major departments in the hospital were represented on the Board, together with two or three union representatives and two or three GPs. They took decisions without having to consult local authorities etc, and trusted Mr Ross and Miss Paton to look after day to day affairs. This was all so much better than the modern, never ending management by committee and consultation.
>
> There was a good atmosphere at Bangour and we all worked happily together with few petty rivalries.

After the coming of the National Health Service, staff from the Plastic Surgery unit at Bangour became responsible for running clinics from the Borders of Scotland to Inverness in the Highlands. All the time the intention was to transfer the unit to Edinburgh and because of this the department always kept its records separate from those of the rest of Bangour General Hospital. Even in 1991, it is still not clear where the long term future of the unit lies. The years passed, however, and the 1950s gave way to the 1960s with the unit still in its original, unsatisfactory premises. In the end this provoked Mr Wallace to threaten that he would no longer be responsible for the welfare of burns patients unless a properly built and equipped burns unit was opened. His dream was eventually realised on 25 June 1968 but at the same time there was disappointment as the following day's *Scotsman* reported:

> A new £66,500 intensive care unit—one of the most advanced in the world for the treatment of severe burns—was opened at Bangour General Hospital, West Lothian, yesterday, by the Very Rev Dr R Leonard Small.
>
> But the twelve bed unit, considered 'a very welcome improvement' to the plastic surgery service of the South Eastern Region, is unlikely to receive any patients for another two months because of a shortage of trained staff. A team of twenty-eight doctors, nurses and medical technicians, fully trained in the skilled operation of an intensive care burns unit, is required and as yet only about half are available.
>
> 'Unless we have a devoted staff at the unit we will achieve nothing and the work and strain is such that we need a large team. Providing a team means the redeployment of certain trained staff and this task will take us a little time,' said Mr A B Wallace, senior consultant at the hospital's plastic surgery and burns unit.
>
> He added, 'As we draw our patients from all over the region a twelve bed unit is not nearly large enough because burning is a much too common accident. Unfortunately we just do not have the staff to cope.
>
> Opening the unit, Dr Small, a former Moderator of the General Assembly of the Church of Scotland (previously a Minister in Bathgate, and whose son, Dr Colin Small, is presently a Consultant Anaesthetist in the hospital) said he hoped it would not only improve the treatment of burns, but also lead to advances in medical knowledge, especially in the field of skin grafts. It is intended to establish a skin bank at the unit. . . .
>
> It is an extension and development of the burns unit which was started when Bangour was built as a war time emergency medical service hospital.
>
> Most of the armed forces' burns cases were treated there, including those from Coastal Command, survivors from the Narvik raid on Norway and the rear gunner who was the sole survivor of the Duke of Kent's plane when it crashed in Sutherland.
>
> The new unit combines the sophisticated with the simple, and some of the equipment is experimental.
>
> There is a monitoring system that can give a continuous indication of heart rate and temperature for each patient both at their bedside and at a central console in the nurses' station.
>
> There is also an experimental surgical dressings-operating table invented by Mr T W Flynn, an operating theatre charge nurse at

Bangour. It allows, for the first time, a severely burned patient to be bandaged without any lifting or turning movements which at present present a problem for theatre staff.

Mr Flynn's invention later brought another little bit of fame to Bangour as it was featured on BBC television's well-known science programme, 'Tomorrow's World'.

Inevitably over the years many of the patients dealt with at Bangour have also hit the headlines because of the spectacular nature of the accidents which have resulted in their coming to the Burns Unit. In some cases patients have even been flown from abroad to Bangour as was the case recently with two teenagers very seriously injured in a gas explosion in a Spanish holiday flat, as Mr Batchelor recalls.

The girls were well treated by the Spanish hospital staff who had gained much experience of burns only a year earlier when a petrol tanker exploded. It was obvious, however, that the girls would require many months of hospital treatment and that it would be much better

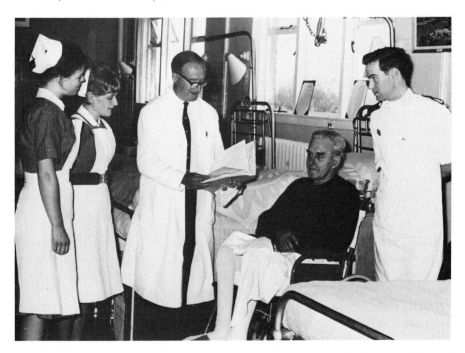

Fig. 43   A B Wallace, famous for his innovative developments in the care of burns' victims, conducts a ward round with Charge Nurse Flynn whose special bed, designed to enable burns' dressings to be changed more easily, was featured on BBC Television's 'Tomorrow's World'.

for them if this could be provided near their homes. With burns victims you either have to move them very soon after the accident or wait until they have almost recovered and it was therefore decided to fly them back to Scotland. A voluntary air ambulance was summoned from Austria and as soon as the girls were loaded aboard in Spain, preparations began at Edinburgh Airport for their reception. As their plane approached, all other traffic was cleared from the area and within seconds of them touching down ambulances accompanied by police out-riders raced across the tarmac to collect them and rush them equally quickly to Bangour. Their treatment proved successful and they still return from time to time so that minor improvements may be made.

In other cases patients have been flown direct to Bangour by helicopter but on the night most recently when Bangour was on stand by, expecting many helicopters to land, none came. That was the night of the Piper Alpha Oil Rig disaster in the North Sea. The emergency medical services in Aberdeen used a pre-arranged system to notify Bangour Burns Unit of the extent of the accident out in the North Sea and all necessary emergency staff responded immediately but sadly there were no survivors for them to treat. The same was true on the night of the Lockerbie air tragedy.

Most of the Burns Unit patients are, unfortunately epileptics who suffer injury during a convulsion, the elderly and confused, or people who have had accidents as a result of drinking or smoking, or a combination of the two. Sadly, fireworks and chip pans also continue to contribute to the toll despite all the warnings about the need for great care with their use. Three recent victims of chip pan fires have been a local general practitioner and two well-known Edinburgh surgeons.

It was in 1944 that one of Bangour's great characters William Donald MacLennan, first came on the scene as acting house surgeon (medical) in the Maxillo-facial, Plastic Surgery and Burns Unit at a salary, per year, of £270—less £100 for board and lodging.

The Plastic Surgery Unit was housed in T1–8 and enjoyed a healthy rivalry with its sister unit at Ballochmyle Hospital in Ayrshire. In the early days Sir Harold Gillies visited these Units in an advisory capacity and his Sunday morning meetings, attended by as many of the staff as were available, were memorable. Cases were discussed, treatment plans evolved, criticism was made no matter how harsh—all designed to ensure improvements in patient care. Sir Harold was a prima donna, an eccentric whose experience was highly valued and which fully justified the worldwide reputation which he enjoyed.

Mr MacLennan's first stay at Bangour only lasted three months as he joined the Royal Naval Volunteer Reserve where he served as a Surgeon Lieutenant until January 1948, when he returned to Bangour as a Registrar (Dental) subsequently becoming Senior Registrar in 1949. Initially he was resident in the old farm house, now sadly demolished. This was a happy hunting ground for at least two of the nursing sisters!

> Bangour was a fascinating place in these days. The staff worked hard and played hard. Cricket in the summer was one of the leisure activities enjoyed by many, the team representing a wide cross section of hospital employees including Jock Milne (general surgeon), myself (oral surgery), Bill Murray (chest physician), Thirkell the head gardener and Osborne the butcher. The wicket was at the Village Hospital. On one occasion Jock Milne was called to an emergency and one of the Village Hospital patients was co-opted to field on the boundary. This created a problem as on the first occasion on which he was called to field the ball he promptly put it in his pocket and steadfastly refused to return it. Scoring in these circumstances left much to be desired.

In 1949 Dr MacLennan went to New York for six months study as a Visiting Scholar and Research Fellow in the Dental School of Columbia University and the Plastic Surgery Service at the Presbyterian Hospital. He was accompanied by his wife whom he had married earlier during his 'active service' in New York.

By the time he returned to Scotland the National Health Service was well established and the prefabricated unit at 'T' block, despite its many shortcomings, was a busy functional unit. The corridors from ward to theatre were open to the winter winds, rain and snow and the patients in transit had to be well covered with blankets. Over the subsequent years progressive improvements were made to fabric and equipment. These were essential in the light of the unexpectedly extended life of the Emergency Medical Services buildings and the increasing patient load. The vastly improved theatre and ward facilities, the new custom built Burns Unit and the general upgrading were most welcome. The Burns Unit was designed to be an infection free area with controlled circulation of air—the great merits of fresh air and open windows lost the day in pursuit of progress.

The development of the entire Oral, Maxillo-facial, Plastic Surgery and Burns Unit led to national and international recognition and the team approach, encouraged by A B Wallace who had been appointed a Commander of the British Empire (CBE), saw members of the staff studying abroad and introducing new concepts on their return. Workshop extensions and a Photographic Department adjacent to the museum and lecture room assisted in furthering the undergraduate, postgraduate and nursing teaching. The name Desmond Franklin will long be remembered in the Photography Department. The 'team' philosophy embraced every member of the staff both lay and professional. Everyone contributed to the happy atmosphere which existed throughout the entire hospital and helped it survive, even when the going was tough.

In 1953 Dr MacLennan was appointed Consultant Dental Surgeon and Honorary Lecturer in Oral Surgery at Edinburgh University, later to become Honorary Senior Lecturer and in 1978 Professor in the first Chair in Oral Surgery.

The scope of work for oral surgery was both extensive and challenging. In addition to the routine dental work with splints for facial fractures, dentures, etc, the workshop undertook provision of items such as hand splints, artificial appliances to replace eyes, ears, noses, and implants for skull defects.

Having been born with one ear, Professor MacLennan was quick to appreciate that reconstructive surgery was not always the ideal answer for people with deformities. He himself had never resorted to surgery as he felt, quite rightly, that to do so would have denied him the opportunity of participating in contact sports such as rugby football, a sport at which he excelled. His decision did not prevent him from getting into the Royal Navy, as mentioned above, despite the fact that he was also deaf and colour blind. We still went on to win the war and Professor MacLennan went on to have a distinguished career in surgical practice.

I found that being handicapped myself perhaps made it easier for me to relate to others with deformities. I could discuss and counsel

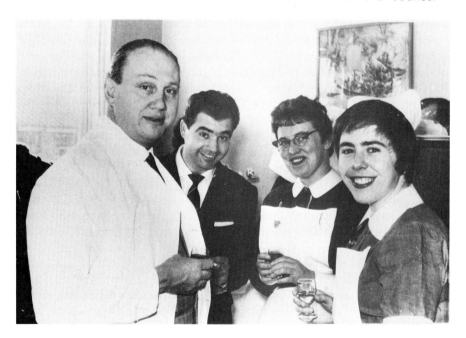

Fig. 44   Bill McLennan entertaining colleagues at a party in 'T' block.

patients more sympathetically, going over the pros and cons of the multiple, lengthy and often stressful courses of treatment.

My duties were not confined to Bangour General Hospital but extended to the Royal Hospital for Sick Children in Edinburgh and clinics in Fife. Throughout my professional life I always believed that surgery was not simply a matter of repetitive cutting. Correct diagnosis is of primary importance, followed by a sound treatment plan for each individual. Undoubtedly there is a place for purely cosmetic surgery as featured in the daily press these days, but one must always realise that all surgery carries with it an inherent risk, however well-intentioned the operator. A young girl was referred to me. She had been bitten on the face by a rat when she was an infant. This led to a unilateral facial deformity and the inability to open her mouth fully, with minor associated problems. An operation to open her mouth was carried out at this time and was successful. She attended at regular intervals thereafter as she grew up. At the age of approximately 15 years she had developed into a most attractive young lady and was increasingly conscious of her appearance. She was worried about the asymmetry of her face and felt that this adversely affected her relationships with eligible young gentlemen. A further operation undertaken to correct her appearance was done with the insertion of a bone graft from her hip. This proved to be technically most rewarding and in some respects far beyond our expectations but alas she did not live to appreciate the improvement—she bled to death. She had developed a factor which prevented her blood from clotting normally—a defect which presents itself in 1 in 1,000,000 cases, and she, regrettably was the unlucky one. This could not have been detected and it is perhaps worth considering whether, with advances in laboratory procedures nowadays, she would have lived. I can still remember acutely that, after our night-long fight to save her life had failed, I walked aimlessly across the fields behind the unit up to the reservoir to try and find the peace of mind that sometimes comes from being alone in such circumstances. On returning to the unit, still clad in my operating clothes, I was convinced that surgery was not for me and I well remember Mr Wallace insisting that I return to the theatre to assist him with his first case of the 'new day'. I have often wondered if he was indicating to me that one must never quit when the going is tough but must learn from one's experiences and go forward again without delay.

At other moments of stress and strain I would go down to the War Memorial Church in the Village Hospital, where I had permission to play the organ. Surrounded by woodcarvings, the handicraft of many patients, and in an atmosphere of tranquillity I could express extremes of emotion playing such tunes as 'By Cool Siloam's Shady Rill' and the 'Pomp and Circumstance March'. Sometimes I was the only person there with the exception of the church cleaners and the odd patient who would appear and sit down on one of the chairs to listen and to meditate. With the everchanging rays of the sun diffusing through the tall windows it was hardly suprising that I found the atmosphere so completely comforting.

I have nothing but happy memories of Bangour—of colleagues and patients with whom I have worked. These will always remain the heart of my work in which I hope I have given a little in return for what I undoubtedly received in plenty. The spirit of camaraderie was an experience never since surpassed, perhaps at its greatest when we all lived in the hospital during those early days of service. We made our own entertainment largely because the town was relatively far away and the last bus home was too early for most of us. In the winter Jock Milne ran regular Scottish Country Dances with Tim Wright and his Broadcasting Band playing on the stage of the Recreation Hall. These and other entertainments were attended by everyone it seemed—doctors, nurses, occupational and physiotherapists, secretaries, even Miss Purdie the Bacteriologist—a well kent figure in 'L' block who, with her physician colleague Miss Helen Gardner, organised the Mess in their own best interests despite frequent opposition from all other occupants who disapproved of their antics. At Christmas we all got together to put on a show. This was eagerly awaited by both patients and staff alike because of the scripts which were liberally punctuated with jokes and local references to all and sundry. Even our own rendering of the Bangour version of 'Juke Box Jury', bearing little or no relationship to the television panel game, was voted a hit. The summer brought cricket, tennis and fishing to the fore. The Annual Hospital Sports Day was a highlight not to be forgotten and the many day and night picnics and 'games' at the reservoir left little or nothing to be desired.

Now that I am retired, living in Gullane, I feel privileged indeed to be able to say in all truth—those were the days.

A current major source of burn injuries is house fires. Many problems in treating these patients arise from the respiratory injuries which they suffer as a result of smoke inhalation, especially when these injuries are caused by fumes from polystyrene foam which is still found in many items of furniture. Again Bangour is pioneering the latest techniques for giving relief to such patients and Senior Anaesthetist Dr Connie Howie and her colleagues have gained unique experience in the relief of their suffering.

Over the years, Bangour Burns Unit has always attracted postgraduate students from aborad including many from the Eastern block countries, especially Czeckoslavakia, and this is still the case today.

As well as burns injuries and the resultant plastic surgery treatments which their wounds require, the unit also deals with many cases of skin cancer and cancers affecting the head and neck. Campbell Buchan is well remembered for the work which he did in these areas of surgical practice during his many years of service to the unit.

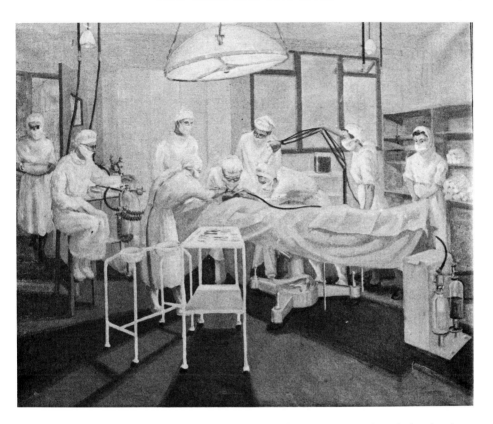

Fig. 45 *Operation in Progress. Scottish Plastic Surgery Unit.* This painting by the artist Eric Rodwell, RSA, 1946, hangs in the library of the Plastic Surgery Unit of Bangour General Hospital.

Dr Jim McLelland, who recently retired as consultant radiotherapist to West Lothian, recalls how referrals to him for treatment of head and neck cancer cases grew from thirty patients in 1957 to over 300 in 1977. At first many of these patients with complicated cancers affecting the head and neck were treated in hospitals in Edinburgh but gradually Bangour developed its own service and was able to deal with all its own cases.

The skill and experience of Bangour's Plastic Surgery department's staff has been recognised much further afield. A B Wallace not only founded the International Society for Burns Injuries, he was also founder and editor of *The British Journal of Plastic Surgery* and a founder member of The British Association of Plastic Surgeons. Three of his colleagues at Bangour have gone on to become its President, including Campbell Buchan, Anne Sutherland and Tony Watson, who holds this post in 1991 and is currently editor of *The British Journal of Plastic Surgery*.

In the 1990s, the department is again among the world leaders in the application of micro surgical techniques. Mr John McGregor took over from Campbell Buchan when he retired in 1981 and, following the retirement of Anne Sutherland and Alastair Batchelor in the late 1980s, two new consultants, Awf Quaba and James Watson joined the unit, bringing new skills with them. Increased collaboration with the orthopaedic surgeons has produced great advances in the care of victims with severe leg and hand injuries. The unit's involvement with the famous breast cancer surgical unit in Edinburgh means that many women now come to Bangour for specialist breast reconstruction after treatment of their cancer.

In October 1989, when most of Bangour General Hospital moved to its new location at St John's Hospital at Howden in Livingston, the Plastic Surgery, Maxillo-facial and Burns Unit was left at the Bangour site and will move down to the new hospital when Phase 2 opens in 1992. Until that date 'T' block in Bangour continues to provide the service to patients from the whole of the south east and the Highlands of Scotland that it has given since the Health Service began in 1948, 43 years ago. Techniques may have changed dramatically and many more patients are admitted than in the old days but they stay in hospital for a much shorter time and there is a continual bustle of activity in the wards and operating theatres. Although much of Bangour is now shuttered and silent, empty except for ghosts and memories, one corner will remain full of life for a little longer. Any of the soldiers treated there during the war nearly fifty years ago would find that they could come back to 'T' block and recognise the old huts in which they spent so many months undergoing treatment.

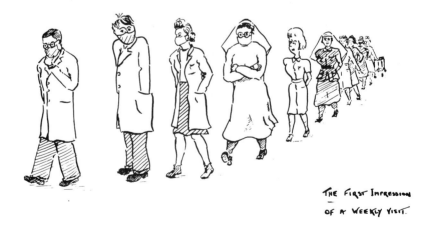

THE FIRST IMPRESSION
OF A WEEKLY VISIT.

David
Blaxill

Chapter Nine

The Bangour Babies—58,329

Bangour General Hospital's Maternity Unit was born at the same time as the infant National Health Service in 1948.

Officially the unit opened on 1 April 1948 but the first baby was actually delivered two days before the opening and, very appropriately, the new arrival was the little daughter of the wife of Bangour's own Consultant General Surgeon, Jock Milne. As it became apparent that the baby's arrival was imminent and was definitely going to beat the official opening of the Bangour Maternity Unit, Mr Milne was said to have been told that he had better get his car out and run his wife, Ina, to hospital in Edinburgh. 'Rubbish,' he is said to have declared, 'either you open the department right away or Ina will just have to have the baby in one of the other wards in 'T' block!' And so Mrs Milne was rushed across from her home in the grounds of the hospital to 'T' block, where the maternity unit was originally housed in T1 and T2, and shortly afterwards baby Linda was delivered safely and became the first of thousands of Bangour babies.

In 1948 most West Lothian mothers had their babies in their own homes, because home deliveries were still the accepted thing in the early post war years. During its first year from Linda's birth on 30 March to 31 December 1948, 275 babies were born at the Bangour Maternity Unit. The women of West Lothian soon grew to appreciate the new service which Bangour offered and during the following year the number of confinements in the new unit grew rapidly, the total number of babies delivered in 1949 reaching 750. Nowadays between 1,700 and 1,800 babies are born in the hospital each year, 1981 being the department's most productive year with 1,898 births. The last baby to be born in the maternity department at Bangour General Hospital was delivered at 6.30 a.m. on the morning of 1 November 1989. He was a healthy 7 lb 5 oz boy called Martin Heggie and was presented with a small silver cup by Dr Ian Brunton, the Senior Obstetrician.

In total, 58,329 babies were born in the maternity unit at Bangour between 30 March 1948 and 1 November 1989, when the department closed with the transfer to St John's Hospital at Howden.

Although Linda Milne was the first baby born in the new maternity unit set up under the equally new National Health Service, she was not the first baby actually to be born at Bangour. For several years immediately after the Second World War, the Polish Army ran a Forces Hospital Unit there and when required, it offered a maternity service for the soldiers' wives. In all 132 successful deliveries took place in the unit. It would be fascinating to know what has happened to these Scottish Poles. This ceased with the official opening of Bangour's Maternity Unit but the Poles decided that a farewell flourish was necessary and, so the story goes, their last maternity patient was therefore delivered by Caesarian section.

The first Consultant in charge of the Bangour Maternity Unit was the late Dr W F T Haultain. He was also in charge of the Gynaecology ward which was at first housed separately across in 'Q' block. In the early 1950s however, the maternity unit was moved to 'S' block and this provided an opportunity to transfer gynae to the neighbouring department where the two services operated happily side by side throughout the remainder of Bangour General Hospital's life span. In 1970–71 extensive upgrading took place in 'S' block and the operating theatre in the department, which had previously been used for both Caesarian sections and gynaecology cases, became purely the gynaecological theatre. A labour ward extension was added to the block to give the unit a very compact but spacious labour suite. It was built to the very highest standards, and included its own Caesarian section theatre. This released accommodation for badly needed office space for secretarial, nursing and medical staff, all of whom had been active participants in the planning of the department.

In the early days of the unit, Ante Natal care was much less detailed than it is now and arrangements for 'shared care' between the hospital, the general practitioner and local midwife were, to say the least, informal. Early on, it was appreciated that access to Bangour General Hospital from the northern part of the county was difficult and in the early 1950s a peripheral Ante Natal clinic was established in Bo'ness, which moved to Linlithgow in the mid 1970s with the reorganisation of Health Board Boundaries when Bo'ness became part of the Forth Valley rather than remaining with the Lothian Health Board. In addition, for the convenience of the patients and as the medical staffing in the unit increased, gynaecological patients were also seen at the clinic.

Bo'ness remained the only out-lying clinic until 1967 when the new town of Livingston was being developed and an experiment in medical care was begun as the brainchild of the late Sir John Brotherston, formerly Chief Medical Officer for Scotland. He was of the opinion that the general practitioners working in Livingston would be interested in training in other specialties in medicine and as a result many of the Livingston general practitioners have had and still hold a dual appointment, combining the role of both a general practitioner and a hospital practitioner working with one of the recognised hospital specialties. The second general practitioner to be appointed to Livingston, Dr Ross Munro, had obstetrics and gynaecology as his particular interest and on his appointment an Ante Natal clinic opened at Craigshill Health Centre in 1968. This was followed in the 1970s by the appointment of Dr Marjory McKinnon to a similar position at Howden Health Centre, and the service has since developed even further. There are now three more Ante Natal clinics for women booked for confinement in Bangour General Hospital, and these are being conducted in Livingston on a regular basis by a combination of dual role general practitioners and hospital doctors. Outside Livingston similar clinics are run by Hospital staff and are held in West Calder and Whitburn. Accordingly, the Hospital Obstetric and Gynaecology Unit services six 'out reach' Ante Natal clinics in West Lothian as well as the three clinics held within the hospital. This wide spread of services reduces travelling problems for the women of West Lothian and as a result the attendance rate at the peripheral Ante Natal clinics is excellent. In addition the distribution of patients to small, out reach Ante Natal clinics allows greater time to be spent on the needs of individual patients and has resulted in close and happy liaison between the community midwives and the hospital staff. This, however, has brought about a significant increase in the work load of the Medical Records Department and the secretaries of the obstetric department, involved in co-ordinating patients' appointments and casenotes.

In the early days of the department the district midwives very often combined midwifery duties with those of district nurse and many also incorporated health visiting duties. These midwives functioned under the auspices of the Local Authorities and the Medical Officer of Health was responsible for them, but in 1974, with the reorganisation of the Health Services, the community midwives in West Lothian became the responsibility of the Senior Nursing Officer for Midwifery Services. Gradually a network of community midwives with duties in defined areas of the West Lothian District became established. These midwives, many of whom trained and worked at Bangour General Hospital, are based in the various Health Centres and work closely with the general practitioners in the provision of Maternity services. In addition they also have close links with the Hospital unit and all midwives have, at regular intervals, to spend some time working in the Hospital unit, in order to keep up to date with those areas of activity outwith the normal duties of the midwife working in the community.

Over the years there have been great changes in the provision of maternity care. Since the 1960s, early discharge from hospital of mother and baby, with the agreement of general practitioner and community midwife, has been a common feature and nowadays is taken for granted. With the introduction of modern techniques such as ultrasound scanning and ante natal diagnosis of some forms of congenital abnormality the complexity and effectiveness of Ante Natal care has increased.

In the labour ward women no longer labour for two, three or even four days, as was frequently the practice thirty or forty years ago, and whereas at one time it was a rare event to see a husband in the labour ward, it is now the rule rather than the exception. In addition, with the assistance and support of the Anaesthetic department, the increased use of epidural anaesthesis has meant that many husbands now choose to be in theatre to be an encouragement to their wives if a child has to be delivered by Caesarian section. The hospital staff, both nursing and medical, have become accustomed to this major change in practice.

The prospective parents of today are infinitely better educated and prepared for parenthood as a result of classes run in hospital by the community midwives and by outside organisations such as the National Childbirth Trust.

Over the years, the gynaecology service has seen a similar change in emphasis with regard to its work patterns. A very significant proportion of gynaecological operating time is nowadays dedicated to aspects of 'population control', or social gynaecology, including terminations of pregnancies and sterilisation. Much of this type of gynaecological practice is undertaken on patients who are only in hospital for one day. This approach has been adopted for most minor gynaecological operations nowadays.

As with patients attending Ante Natal clinics, modern women are very much better informed about gynaecological matters than were their predecessors. However many women and their partners require extensive counselling on certain aspects of gynaecological disease and this is particularly true in cases of infertility. The gynaecologist must be prepared to discuss in detail options open to a woman, and help her come to an informed decision about the best course of action for her particular set of circumstances.

The gynaecology department in Bangour General Hospital has established close links with the highly specialised gynaecological services available in Edinburgh, for the benefit of women in West Lothian who can now seek specialised types of treatments for some causes of infertility, problems of bladder function, management of some types of malignant disease and endocrinological aspects of gynaecology.

The obstetric and gynaecology department in Bangour General Hospital has always had the reputation for being a happy, hard working and informal unit and a lot of credit for this must go to the late Dr Janet Worling. Dr Worling first worked as a resident house officer in the obstetric and gynaecology department of the hospital in the early 1950s. She subsequently returned to Bangour in June 1955 as senior registrar, and remained with the department from then until her death in December 1980. During Dr Worling's eleven years as a Senior Registrar, Dr W D A Callan and the late Dr Donald Irvine were the part-time consultants in the unit, visiting West Lothian from Edinburgh, where they were based. In 1966 Dr Worling was made a consultant and during the years she worked at the Hospital she acquired a reputation for kindliness, common sense, skill and compassion which endeared her to countless colleagues and patients. Such was the esteem in which she was held that, following her death at a relatively early age, a Trust Fund was set up in her memory to provide funding for educational activities for obstetric and gynaecological nursing staff, supplementary to funds provided by the National Health Service. The Trust Fund, which is administered by independent Trustees has proved a great success and has kept alive the memory of Dr Worling.

From the 1950s Edinburgh University medical students have regularly spent time in the unit and many have subsequently returned to work there following graduation. One of the current consultant staff, who wishes to remain anonymous for obvious reasons, as will become apparent, well remembers his first visit to the Caesarian section theatre as a medical student. While assisting at the very first Caesarian section which he had ever seen, the pyjama cord which held his operating theatre trousers up and maintained his dignity, became loose. The only recourse left to him was to lean heavily against the operating table thereby occluding venous return from his legs to his heart and resulting, some several minutes later, in a gradual loss of

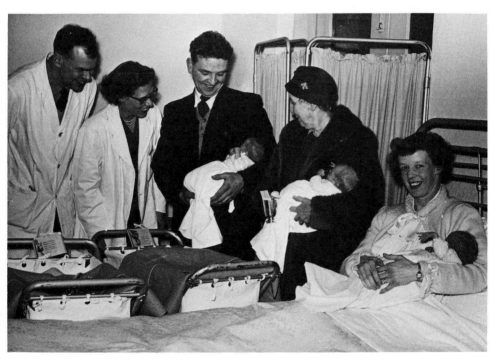

Fig. 46   Dr Janet Worling (second from the left) sharing the joy and pleasure with Mrs McLay and her family after the safe delivery of triplets, 22 February 1957.

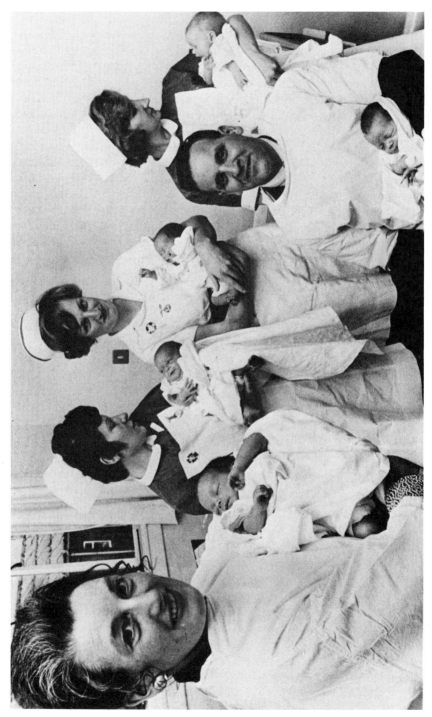

Fig. 47(a) The Bostock quins.

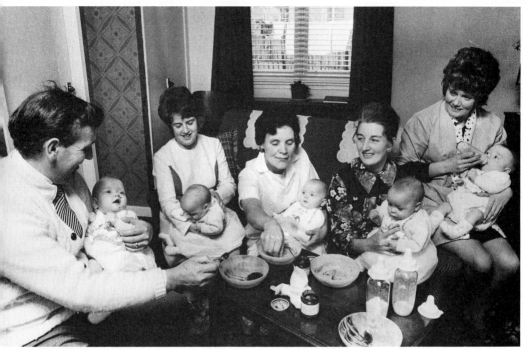

Fig. 47(b)   The problems of feeding five hungry babies at one time.

consciousness. It is recorded, according to folklore, that his trousers hit the floor some 5 seconds before he did!

Fortunately this particular incident never made newspaper headlines, but the safe arrival of Bangour General Hospital's first ever set of triplets did. The *Lothian Courier* reported on 22 February 1957:

> A 26 year old Armadale woman, Mrs Elizabeth McLay, has given birth to triplets in the Maternity Unit at Bangour Hospital. Although the Maternity Unit has been operating since 1948, this is the first occasion that there have been triplets. The boys, who are named Jim and Kenneth, were born between 11 p.m. and midnight on Wednesday and weighed 4 lbs 7 oz and 5 lbs 5 oz respectively. Their sister Janet will celebrate her birthday a day later as she was not born until almost 12.30 a.m. yesterday morning. Janet weighs 4 lbs 15 oz. Mrs McLay already has an 18 month old child who was also born at Bangour.

While the birth of the McLay triplets was reported in the local newspapers in West Lothian, the safe arrival of the Bostock quins on 14 April 1972 was

widely reported in the national press. These quins were naturally occurring—
no fertility drug had been used—and Mrs Bostock had been an in-patient in
the department from the time when the diagnosis of quins was made until
the time of delivery fourteen weeks later. The quins were delivered approximately six weeks prematurely. As far as the hospital staff can discover the
only other record of quintuplets having been delivered in Scotland was early
in the nineteenth century in the North East. These poor babies were about
twelve weeks premature and, not surprisingly in those days, none of them
survived. As well as being a medically unique occasion, therefore, the successful delivery and survival of the Bostock quins was also a very happy one.
Mr and Mrs Bostock received a tremendous amount of support from the
Local Authority, friends and relatives. Their church and faith also provided
them with tremendous courage and it was a pleasing reward for their patience
that the progress of the quins following delivery was so straightforward and
unremarkable. The Bostock quins have grown up as normal children in their
community and have, happily, been spared the pressures and publicity that
are commonly associated with multiple births in this day and age.

The transfer of the obstetric and gynaecology department from Bangour
General Hospital to the new hospital in Livingston opens up even wider
horizons for the development of the unit, as the population in West Lothian
continues to grow, from approximately 100,000 in 1948 to 145,000 in 1989.

Chapter Ten

The Patients Kept Coming

In 1964 Mr Noel Gray and Mr Jock Milne were joined by a third consultant surgeon, Mr A A Gunn, a graduate of the Edinburgh Medical School who had received his surgical training at both the Royal Infirmary and the Western General Hospitals in Edinburgh.

In addition to his special clinical interests in biliary and colon surgery, which were to form the basis of extensive clinical research over the ensuing years, Tony Gunn developed a major programme of study in computer based diagnosis applied to the assessment of patients with abdominal pain. He successfully involved generations of junior colleagues with these programmes during their time as registrars in the general surgical unit in West Lothian. Of equal importance, he developed collaborative studies in the diagnosis and management of abdominal pain with some of the West Lothian general practitioners.

Mr Gunn's clinical research was characterised by meticulous record keeping, allowing him to accumulate accurate information on all his patients but particularly those with gallbladder disease, peptic ulceration and colo-rectal disease. This information formed the basis of a continuous process of audit of his own performance and led to the introduction of technical modifications and innovations. It was also the basis of numerous publications, many involving the surgical registrars, which were largely responsible for the increased recognition of the General Surgical Unit in Bangour as a centre of excellence both in national and international terms. An equally important consequence of Tony Gunn's commitment to audit and his expertise with computerisation was the major contribution he was able to make to the development of the Edinburgh Surgical Audit System. This System, the first of its kind in the United Kingdom, has subsequently been recognised as leading the way in an area which has been perceived as vital to the cost effective deployment of surgical resources.

The stimulating surgical atmosphere in West Lothian created by Noel Gray, Jock Milne and Tony Gunn ensured that the annual Saturday Morning Clinical Surgery Meeting, conducted by Bangour General Hospital on behalf of the Edinburgh University Department of Surgery, was one of the best

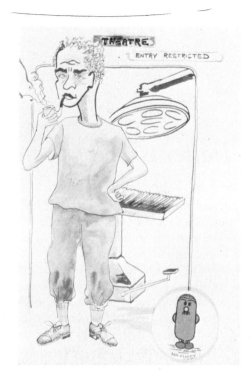

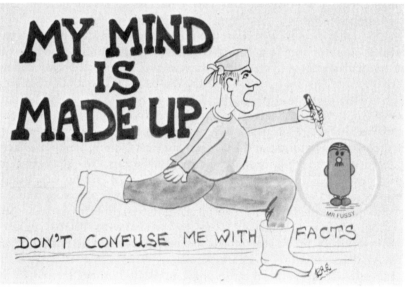

Fig. 48(a) and (b)   Tony Gunn's distinctive personality inspired the cartoonist's pen.

attended by surgical staff from Edinburgh, the Borders and Fife. These meetings were always guaranteed to provoke considerable debate on the challenges offered to many long established surgical rituals.

At the same time as maintaining a very high standard of clinical practice with close personal supervision of the individual patients under his care, Tony Gunn was also actively involved with the Edinburgh Post Graduate Board for Medicine and the Royal College of Surgeons of Edinburgh as a teacher and examiner. As a result of his active support of the Royal College of Surgeons he was elected a Member of the Council of the College. His many other outside commitments included membership of the Editorial Board of the *British Journal of Surgery*.

The stimulating atmosphere of the surgical unit extended into the realm of sport. All three surgeons played golf and Tony Gunn also excelled at squash, challenging all junior staff to a game, while Jock Milne was an enthusiastic tennis player until his accident.

April 1976 saw the retirement of Jock Milne and in October of the same year Noel Gray retired, their posts being filled by Mr Donald Macleod and

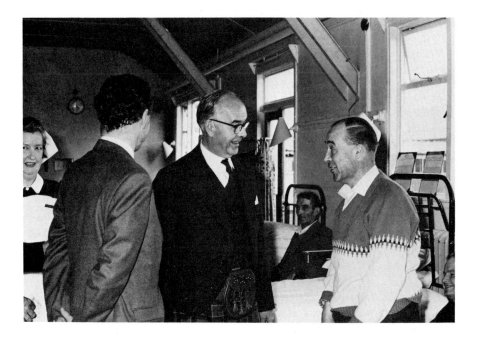

Fig. 49   Lord Harold Birsay visited Bangour General Hospital during his period of office as Lord High Commissioner to the Church of Scotland Annual General Assembly from 1965–66. He visited the surgical wards in 'Q' block accompanied by Sister Christie and Mr Tony Gunn, Consultant Surgeon.

Mr Ian Wallace respectively. Both these new members of the surgical staff in Bangour were Edinburgh graduates and surgical trainees.

Donald Macleod, who had spent a year working in Birmingham and American Trauma Centres, had a particular interest in the management of the injured patient and, until the appointment of an Accident and Emergency Consultant, Dr Peter Freeland in 1989, included clinical and administrative responsibility for the Accident and Emergency Department among his duties. Over and above his commitment to general surgery and the Accident Department, Mr Macleod also had a special interest in sports medicine, holding the appointment of Honorary Medical Adviser to the Scottish Rugby Team when he took up his post in West Lothian and laterally becoming increasingly involved with the Scottish Sports Council and with the provision of medical services at the 13th Commonwealth Games held in Edinburgh in 1986.

Mr Macleod described his association with the Scottish Rugby Team as 'a result of being in the right place at the right time'. He continues:

> In 1966 I was senior house officer working with Professor Sir John Bruce who had been invited to become Honorary Medical Advisor to the Scottish Rugby Union. Sir John had a great love of association football and had been closely involved with Hibernian football club in Edinburgh. He had little or no knowledge or experience of rugby football and invited his senior lecturer, Mr J W W Thomson and myself to make all the necessary arrangements. My commitment gradually developed from that time and the first match at which I was the team doctor, sitting at the side of the International pitch at Murrayfield, was in 1969 when Scotland was, unfortunately, beaten by Ireland. Jim Telfer, MBE, was captain of the Scottish Rugby Team for that game and had to be replaced because he had sustained concussion.
>
> The involvement of doctors in rugby football has increased significantly since that time and, in many respects, Scotland has led the way. I have been lucky enough to be a member of the Medical Advisory Committee to the International Rugby Football Board since its inception in 1978 and was chosen to accompany the Scottish Rugby Team on its tour in New Zealand in 1981 and 1990 and I also visited that country as doctor to the British Lions Rugby Touring Team in 1983.

Mr Noel Gray had included among his interests the surgery of the urinary tract and this was reflected in the appointment of his successor, Ian Wallace, as a general surgeon with a special interest in urology. Following his appointment Mr Wallace developed the management of surgery of the urinary tract at a time when there has been a steady increase in new technology, replacing open operations on the kidney, ureter, bladder and prostate with much less invasive endoscopic techniques.

Surgery in the 1970s and 1980s was characterised by a movement towards increased specialisation following the realisation that the development of a relatively limited field of surgical expertise by an individual or small group of surgeons was associated with better results. While certain fields of surgery had already developed clearly defined specialities, such as neurosurgery, which had started in the south east of Scotland with Professor Dott working at Bangour Hospital, the traditional 'General Surgeon' was still a common phenomenon at the beginning of this period. This was particularly true in hospitals such as Bangour where the three consultants had provided a broadly based surgical service particularly with regard to emergencies and accidents. A major step forward in the care of accident victims was the appointment in 1975 of a consultant orthopaedic surgeon, Mr James Christie, albeit initially on a part-time basis. It was not until 1980 that a complete orthopaedic service was established, freeing the general surgeon from responsibility for the care of patients with fractures and other orthopaedic problems.

James Christie recalls:

It seemed to be just my luck that the consultant post that I wished to apply for was advertised at a time when I was working in California. The first problem was to get my application form back to Edinburgh before the closing date and the second was to find enough cash to fly home for the interviews. $856 was no mean sum for an overseas surgical trainee working in the United States in the mid 1970s! The bank manager in Nord Hoff, Los Angeles refused my request for a loan despite every imprecation known to man. Curiously enough, help came from an American family who had become great friends. They had been reduced to great penury by the American system of medicine when both their daughters had contracted poliomyelitis at the same time. Tragically one of the girls died and the other was left seriously paralysed. Despite the usual private health care insurance policies, the parents had been forced to make enormous financial sacrifices and their dream was of a national system of health provision free at the point of delivery. They said many times that they would like to see a system similar to the Health Service in Britain and they were more than pleased to offer temporary financial assistance to me.

I had worked in Bangour as a registrar in 1969 and required no persuading of the excellence of its clinical services. My American friends working in their fabulous medical centre had never been exposed to the threat of invasion during the Second World War and were more than interested to see pictures of the hutted hospital to which I would return and not all their comments were complimentary. It still interests and delights me to this very day that at least twice as much work seemed to be done in those huts and it was carried out to just as high a standard as in the palaces of high technology that seemed to cost so much to build and run.

There had been no orthopaedic surgeon at Bangour before my arrival so out patient clinics, fracture clinics and so forth had all to be set up. My plan at that time was to develop a complete, integrated orthopaedic service on site and it was necessary to plan and build the orthopaedic wards and an orthopaedic operating theatre. The operating theatres available at that time in 'Q' block had many features which made them unsuitable for modern orthopaedic procedures such as joint replacement. The operating theatres were shared with the general surgeons and did not have any form of controlled ventilation considered necessary to ensure that the air reaching an orthopaedic operating theatre was free of any bacteria. 'Q' block theatres had no air conditioning at all and became almost unbearably hot on some summer days. Happily the windows could be opened and, so long as someone stood guard with a fly spray or swat, one could continue operating in relative comfort with a pleasant view of the surrounding countryside and grazing cattle or sheep, something that is denied to us nowadays in our modern windowless operating theatres. Unfortunately my request for a specialist orthopaedic theatre to be built was rejected and it became necessary to transfer all major elective and some complex traumatic orthopaedic cases into Edinburgh.

Before my arrival, fractures, and some aspects of orthopaedic surgery had been undertaken by my general surgical colleagues and I have nothing but admiration for the way in which they looked after an enormous number of patients with every kind of problem.

Specialisation brings with it changes and inevitably things begin to cost more. The instruments in use at the time of my arrival in Bangour were so old that no one knew where they had come from or when they had been purchased. I suspect that most of the equipment was pre World War Two and considerably out of fashion although it remained perfectly serviceable. One item of equipment was particularly exciting and had been gifted during World War Two by an American Regiment some thirty years earlier. At that time patients with fractures of the hip required a specialist operating table and you may imagine my surprise and delight on setting up theatre to undertake such an operation, when an enormous piece of historic equipment was produced with the 'Shropshire Horse' engraved on a brass plate along its side! I spent many hours happily in the company of that table putting together a variety of complex fractures entirely successfully and I am only sorry to report that its eventual successor proved to be far less worthy.

My arrival in West Lothian sadly meant that Mr Willie Anderson, consultant orthopaedic surgeon who conducted paediatric out patient orthopaedic clinics in West Lothian, had finally reached retiral age. I soon found out that many of his devoted patients were to treat his youthful replacement with considerable suspicion, particularly as my advice frequently contradicted his own, reflecting a general change in modern orthopaedic philosophy. 'Whit's happened tae Mr Onderson?'

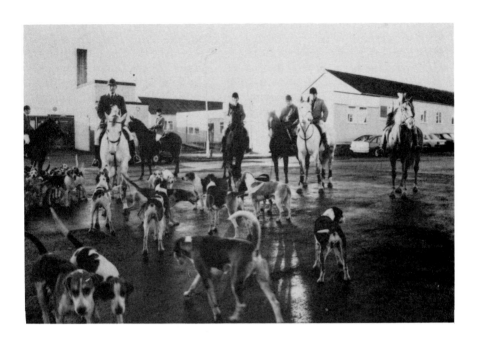

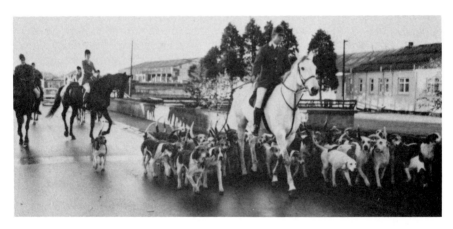

Figs. 50 and 51   One of the views from Bangour's windows. The Linlithgow and Stirlingshire Hunt traditionally hunted the covert wood at Bangour and their arrival was of major interest, especially to long-stay patients. Many a ward round faded into insignificance as the hunt passed through the hospital grounds.

As a special dispensation in 1989, to mark the impending closure of Bangour General Hospital, the hunt, under its Master Mr Coward, paid one last visit.

meant that my opinion did not enjoy much of what my daughter would call 'street cred'! 'Yer offy young, son' was even worse. Mr Anderson had been the first resident house doctor in the Princess Margaret Rose Orthopaedic Hospital and undoubtedly inspired tremendous confidence among his patients—one of the great gifts of healing. He is still missed by his old patients who recognised a kindred spirit in him for he too had suffered orthopaedic illness during his youth and had a special interest in children's problems. Indeed he was for many years the main stay of the paediatric orthopaedic service in the district clinics in West Lothian.

It did not take long after my appointment in 1975 for the work of the newly created orthopaedic unit to get into manageable routine. The enthusiasm of the nursing and other ward staff, indeed all involved in the service, made it all seem relatively easy. If my colleagues in general surgery resented the intrusion of an orthopaedic service they did not at any time give the slightest indication of this and were incredibly kind, allowing invasion of their ward space, theatre time and out patient clinics. My ambition was that there should be an orthopaedic unit in Bangour as good as the general surgical department established by Noel Gray, Jock Milne and Tony Gunn.

Recently, in 1989, I was reading the *Times* newspaper and was delighted to read a large centre page article devoted to the merits of the computer audit system for surgery developed by Tony Gunn at Bangour Hospital. My colleagues were excellent surgeons and remarkable characters; I well remember looking up in the midst of some tricky operative procedure one day to find one of my seniors peering over my shoulder, wearing his golfing clothes and holding a red handkerchief across his mouth instead of the normal theatre gown and mask. 'Just looking in to see what you are doing,' he would say. There were endless lectures too, in a broad Kincardineshire accent, describing the feeding habits of suckler pigs so that one began to wonder if there was a special link between farming and surgery. There is no doubt that I joined a happy and productive surgical unit and it was a privilege to be able to help establish the orthopaedic services in West Lothian.

There have been many changes in the orthopaedic service in Bangour Hospital since it was initially established in 1975. In 1979 I moved to Edinburgh and Mr Jon Cochrane was appointed as the principal consultant providing orthopaedic services in West Lothian. Subsequently the service developed to such an extent that several consultant surgeons, including Mr Michael McMaster, Mr Malcolm McNicol and Mr Jeff Hooper, spent short periods in West Lothian before taking up full-time appointments in Edinburgh. At the time that the orthopaedic unit closed in Bangour Hospital Mr Jon Cochrane was working with Mr Ian Annan and Miss Margaret McQueen as the orthopaedic team providing a comprehensive service for West Lothian, working in conjunction with the Princess Margaret Rose Hospital in Edinburgh.

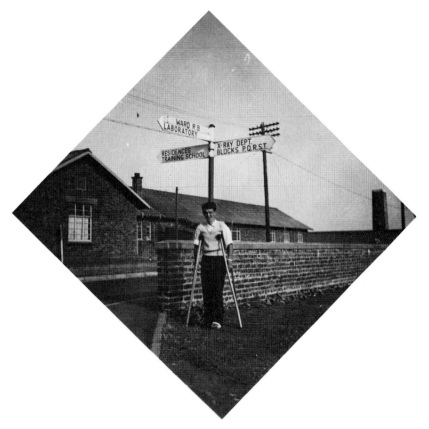

Fig. 52 This patient, recovering from a broken leg, enjoys a walk to the main crossroads in the General Hospital.

I have no doubt that Scottish patients are the best in the world and deserve the very best treatment. I sometimes think that they are too stoical and do not complain enough, even when there is just cause, but of course that is what makes them the very best patients. Patients like that require the very best in the way of treatment and all of us involved in the Health Service hope that this is what we have established for the people in West Lothian in the orthopaedic department.

In addition to the establishment of urological and orthopaedic services in West Lothian, careful audit of the results of vascular surgery led in 1980 to an agreement with the specialist vascular surgeons in Edinburgh that patients requiring this type of surgery would in future be transferred there. This decision coincided with a general recognition that vascular surgery had developed into a separate speciality rather than being part of the function of general surgery.

During this period of change and development in surgical practice the Bangour Unit underwent dramatic transformation in its junior staffing and involvement in Surgical Training. In 1964 the staff consisted of two consultants, a registrar and two house officers, looking after approximately 102 surgical beds. By 1980 the full development of a separate orthopaedic unit meant the general surgical bed complement had been reduced to ninety, under the care of three consultants, three registrars, a senior house officer and five house surgeons. The registrars were part of a three-year rotational training programme involving Edinburgh, and the senior house officers participated in the two-year rotation based in Bangour General Hospital but including experience in plastic surgery, burns and accident and emergency.

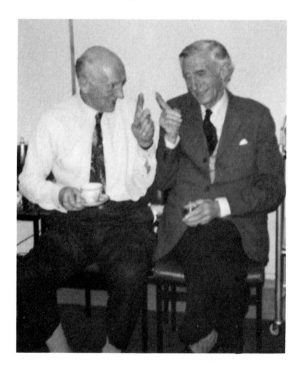

Fig. 53 Retirement. Jock Milne (left) and Noel Gray worked together as Consultant Surgeons for almost thirty years, providing surgical and accident services in Bangour General Hospital and West Lothian for twenty years before they were joined by Mr A A Gunn in 1964. They retired six months apart in 1976, and are captured here in a typical pose—full of life with Jock looking forward to farming, playing cards and lively discussions on every aspect of life, while Noel was planning regular visits to Bruntsfield Golf Club, where he was elected Captain during 1977–79.

Further involvement with the Edinburgh Surgical Training programmes came in 1984 when Bangour was included in the senior registrar training rotations. This involvement of the Unit in senior house officer, registrar and senior registrar training programmes came about as a result of widespread recognition that the quality of experience available in the Surgical Unit at Bangour Hospital was outstanding.

In 1988 Mr Tony Gunn retired, although he continued his connections with the Royal College of Surgeons in Edinburgh in the role of Honorary Librarian. His replacement was Mr John Rainey, an Ulster-born Edinburgh Medical Graduate and Surgical Trainee whose special interest lay in endoscopic surgery of the gastrointestinal and biliary tract as well as colorectal surgery. He had developed these skills in Edinburgh, Bristol and London. These clinical interests are complimented by an active commitment to medical audit.

Over the years the senior staff of the Surgical Unit, starting with Noel Gray and Jock Milne before they retired in 1976, had been involved in the planning of the new hospital in Livingston which was eventually to replace Bangour. Much discussion, some of it acrimonious, took place concerning issues such as the design of the operating theatres, the provision of accident and emergency facilities, the design and provision of intensive care areas, high dependency units and the lay out of the wards. Eventually general surgery, urology and orthopaedic units with all accident and emergency services were transferred to St John's Hospital at Howden on 28 October 1989 thus ending fifty years of service by 'Q' block to the patients of West Lothian.

THE MEDICAL UNIT

In the first forty years of the Hospital, the Medical Unit provided a general medical service. Dr Alistair Wright was the first General Physician to be appointed. Later he was joined by Dr Joyce Grainger. Dr Wright achieved distinction at local and national levels by being elected Vice-President of the College of Physicians of Edinburgh and later a member of the General Medical Council. Dr Grainger was, for many years, a member of the Council of the College of Physicians of Edinburgh. She was also active in developing undergraduate and postgraduate teaching at Bangour. Many overseas doctors have memories of their stay, particularly in cold, snowy winters.

Gradually increasing specialisation has seen the introduction of respiratory medicine, cardiology, diabetes and endocrinology. The first medical subspecialty to develop was respiratory medicine. With the effective control of tuberculosis by Dr Summers and his colleagues, it was possible to extend the service to include other respiratory diseases. Dr Kelman Robertson was a

Physician at the Royal Infirmary in the 1960s and visited Bangour where he developed a special interest in the health problems of coal miners. In due course this led to the setting up, by the Coal Board, of the Institute of Occupational Medicine in Edinburgh which continues to undertake research in the field of industrial hazards. Away from hospital work, Dr Summers and a number of his colleagues were active members of the Edinburgh Medical Curling Club. This club, established in 1912, played regularly at the old Haymarket Ice Rink until 1979, and now at Murrayfield and Gogar Park. George Summers skipped rinks for many years acquiring an awesome reputation for his method of showing displeasure at the poor shots of his team—he would turn his back to the speeding stone, ignoring its progress. Other members of staff from Bangour Hospitals played regularly, including Sir Walter Mercer, Robert Saffley and Ken Wood, Jock Milne and more recently the present Secretary of the Club, John Irving. Ken Wood, consultant radiologist, had the distinction of winning the 'Points' Cup with 40 points in 1976 (world record 44 points). When Dr Summers retired, his successor, Dr Kenneth Murray, and his colleague, Dr Gordon Robertson, were faced with the challenging transition from the apparently narrow field of tuberculosis to the full range of respiratory and other general medical conditions. Dr Wilson Middleton, who succeeded Dr Murray in 1977, has continued to develop the service, having a particular interest in asthma, lung cancer and occupational lung diseases. It is noteworthy that Dr Middleton's secretary, Mrs Margaret Strachan, has been personal secretary to successive Consultants in the Chest Unit since 1953. Her outstanding service was recently acknowledged by the Lothian Health Board when she was presented with the Chairman's Award.

In cardiovascular disease, the most common condition is coronary artery disease. Coronary Care Units were developed in the 1960s. The Unit in Bangour opened in 1972 and now admits approximately 650 patients per year. Technical support from medical physics technician, Bob Duncan, and from ECG technicians, Mae Urquhart, Cameron Slorach and Dorothy Livingstone, has been an important part of service provision as diagnostic techniques become more sophisticated. The Lothian Health Board and locally generated funds have been able to provide the necessary equipment such as cardiac ultrasound, ECG monitors and x-ray imaging to complement the clinical service. Coronary Care Units are successful, thanks mainly to the training and care of nursing staff. In the last ten years there has been continuity of staff. Maureen Smith, a fanatical Aberdeen Football Club supporter, came from London in 1980 to be Sister in the Unit and since then has been helped by many staff, too numerous to mention by name. The immediate care of the patient after a heart attack must now be followed by active rehabilitation. Fortunately the Physiotherapy Department has been able to provide a programme for out-patients, much appreciated by the patients, to improve their

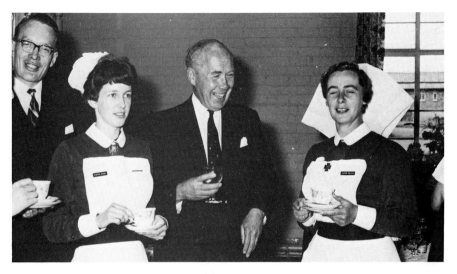

Fig. 54   Dr Alistair Wright, Consultant Physician, is enjoying the company of Sister Grieve, to his left, at a reception. Dr Henry Turner, in the background, is sharing in the fun of the occasion.

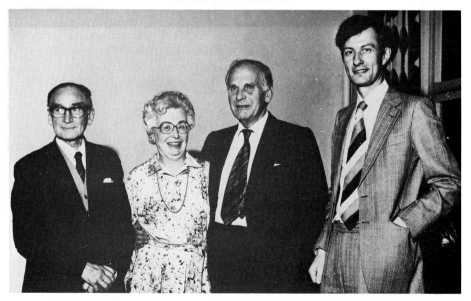

Fig. 55   Dr George Summers was succeeded by Dr Kenneth Murray, on the left, who retired in 1977 after spending the greater part of his professional life looking after patients with tuberculosis and other chest diseases. At his retiral he was joined by Dr Joyce Grainger, Dr Gordon Robertson and Dr Wilson Middleton (on the right) who, in turn, succeeded Dr Murray.

confidence after a serious illness. In 1970 patients would spend three weeks in hospital after a heart attack. Now, the average is five days. Much of this progress is due to the leadership of Dr John Irving.

The Medical Unit has further expanded its sub-specialties by the provision of a special diabetic clinic, initiated by Dr Grainger and expanded by Dr Stuart Gray. Dr Gray's expertise in other less common but nevertheless complex endocrine disorders has been invaluable. More recently Dr Bob Will and Dr Nigel Hurst, visiting consultants from Edinburgh, have set up specialist clinics in Neurology and Rheumatology respectively. As described elsewhere, services for the elderly were initially developed by Dr Bill Conacher. The service has been expanded further and is now fully integrated within the Medical Unit. The challenge of coping with this ever increasing demand has been taken by enthusiastically by Dr John Wilson and his recently appointed colleague, Dr Donald Farquhar.

EAR, NOSE AND THROAT SERVICES IN WEST LOTHIAN

Ear, Nose and throat surgery in the Lothians was founded as a special service in the 1880s when two wards off the medical corridor in the Royal Infirmary of Edinburgh were designated purely for this type of surgery. It is still a unique tradition in Edinburgh that ear, nose and throat surgeons are called 'doctor' as opposed to the more usual term for a surgeon which is 'mister'.

It was in the early 1950s that ear, nose and throat services were first begun in Bangour Village Hospital. Initially it was a purely out patient service but with the move to Bangour General Hospital in 1959 a full service of inpatient beds and an operating theatre reserved for this specialty was established. The original site was 'P' block. The out patient clinic and the surgeons changing room subsequently became the medical library when the department moved to 'R' block. At that time surgery consisted mainly of the management of infection. Acute streptococcal mastoiditis was common place and one of the most frequently performed operations was the Schwatz mastoidectomy to drain pus from the mastoid bone. Other operations included straightforward nose operations such as submucus resection of a deviated nasal spetum, adenoidectomy and tonsillectomy. Tonsillectomy was usually carried out, especially in children, by encircling the tonsil with a metal instrument called a guillotine, which incorporated a hole just large enough to encircle the tonsil, which was then trapped in position with a metal shutter and the tonsil removed by twisting the instrument while at the same time dissecting the tonsil away from the throat with the forefinger of the opposite hand. Using this technique, removal of both tonsils and adenoids would take in the region of 20 seconds. Previously this procedure had been carried out on 'the kitchen table', but improved standards of care in hospital added considerably to the safety of the procedure. Ear, nose and throat surgeons are still endearingly called 'tonsil twisters' by their colleagues in other specialties.

The consultants working in Bangour as well as Edinburgh at that time were Drs Farquharson and McDowell and they operated on approximately 1,000 patients a year. The theatre sister's name was Miss Ferguson and the junior doctor was Dr McQuarrie.

Ear, nose and throat surgery has advanced significantly over the last thirty years, with the development of operating microscopes and specialist lighting allowing the surgeon to peer into the deep dark recesses of the ear, nose and throat. The operation of fenestration to relieve deafness due to otosclerosis was begun in the early 1950s and one of the youngest patients at that time to have this procedure carried out was Miss Margaret Reid, now Mrs Marshall, when she was 16 years old. (Margaret subsequently trained as a nurse at Bangour and was the gold medallist in her year.) This operation was a demanding technique which required considerable skill on the part of the surgeon and the fact that Mrs Marshall retains excellent hearing to this day stands testament to the expertise of the surgery she received. This operation was later replaced by Stapes mobilisation in which the small stirrup bone (Stapes) which had become stiffened is released. Subsequently the operation of stapedectomy was developed in the late 1950s and introduced to Bangour as the treatment of choice for this particular type of deafness.

Sister Ferguson was replaced as theatre sister in the ear, nose and throat department by Sister Chalmers and the sister in charge of the wards at that time was Miss Purves. The first registrar in the department was Arnold Grier, who has only recently retired in Inverness. In 1957 Joe Brown, who has become a legend in his own time, was appointed charge nurse to the ear, nose and throat theatre and clinic and co-ordinated the move from 'P' to 'R' block. Philip Stell was registrar and he has since become one of the most eminent ear, nose and throat surgeons in the world. He is Professor of Otolaryngology in Liverpool. In 1958 Dr Farquharson, who also worked in the Fife hospitals, brought patients from Fife to Bangour for their surgery because the service in West Lothian was considered to be highly efficient.

In the 1960s there was a rather unsettled period during which there were several changes in the consultant staff but the most notable appointment was that of Dr Brian Dale who replaced Dr Farquharson. Dr Dale built up and expanded the surgical repertoire in the ear, nose and throat department in West Lothian, introducing a wide range of microscopic ear operations including myringoplasty and tympanoplasty in which bones of the middle ear are reconstituted to improve hearing.

Recent additions to the consultant staff in West Lothian are Dr Waryam Singh and Dr John Murray, who continue to have dual appointments in Edinburgh. In addition to the area of clinical practice already identified, ear, nose and throat surgery has increasingly become involved in the treatment of head and neck cancer.

When Dr Waryam Singh came to work in the Ear, Nose and Throat Department of Bangour General in 1980, he initiated a programme of research in the field of restoration of speech after surgery of the larynx, the success of which resulted in the highly successful international voice symposium being held at the hospital between 12 and 14 August 1987, the first time that Bangour General Hospital had hosted a major international research conference.

During the early 1980s Dr Singh carried out many successful operations on patients with cancer of the larynx. The lives of these patients were saved but their voices were lost. The only hope of speech in those days was six months of exhaustive therapy, during which time attempts were made to teach them how to swallow mouthfuls of air and then make sounds by belching it up in a controlled manner. This involved the patient placing a finger over a hole in the front of the throat. The patient found the whole procedure extremely difficult and very embarrassing with the result that only about one-third of the patients who had their larynx removed (including the famous British film actor, Jack Hawkins) succeeded in recovering any power of speech.

Dr Singh was very distressed that he could not offer patients a better and more successful operation designed to cure their cancer as well as allowing them the opportunity of speech after the operation. Accordingly, he initiated a programme of research in the course of which he recognised that the whole of the larynx was not cancerous in many patients and that by skillful use of precise microscopic surgery he could safely leave the back wall of the larynx untouched by his operation. This then allowed him to form a flap of skin tissue which enabled air from the lungs to be used by the patients to make sounds instead of having to swallow air and then regurgitate it to assist speech.

By this time, patients from far beyond the Bangour catchment area were coming to Dr Singh for operations on the larynx and he found that using this method many patients could say their first words within eight to ten days of the operation. However, it was still necessary for the patients to control the sounds which they made by inserting one of their fingers into the lower part of their trachea or windpipe. This caused considerable embarrassment to both the patients and the people to whom they were speaking. In addition, Dr Singh felt that this procedure was very unhygienic. Once again he started a series of experiments and one day noticed a small plastic valve which his Anaesthetist was using and asked if he might have the ones from used gas cylinders. He took these valves home and the first valve for insertion in a patient's throat was perfected on his kitchen table.

The use of valves completely revolutionalised the degree to which patients could recover their speech, particularly as Dr Singh was able to identify those words which could readily be pronounced correctly and those which caused difficulty. At this stage, to assist in his work, Dr Singh was able to establish a voice research laboratory adjacent to the Ear, Nose and Throat clinic. At first Dr Singh worked single-handedly often returning home after a long day of operating to work late into the night. Gradually news of his successes spread and the Scottish Home and Health Department provided its first ever research grant to the Ear, Nose and Throat department of a general hospital to allow Dr Singh to employ his first assistant. Subsequent grants have permitted him to extend the staff in his Voice Research Laboratory to include Speech Scientist, Dr W A Ainsworth, Research Fellow, Gordon McKenna, and Speech Therapist, Gary Withnell. Dr Singh was the first to pay tribute to the devoted work of his small team and the great assistance he has received from Charge Nurse Joe Brown working in the out patient clinics and the operating theatres.

Funding for this pioneering work has been assisted by many patients, grateful friends, ranging from a cheque of £100, sent in by a group of appreciative workmates to the thousands of pounds that have been raised by the Laryngectomy Club which was formed by former patients in 1983. In addition to its fund raising role, Dr Singh greatly values the tremendous support which the Laryngectomy Club gives to new patients. 'Hearing for themselves how very successfully former patients can speak has been the very best tonic of all to patients undergoing cancer surgery on their throat', comments Dr Singh. For Waryam Singh himself, the entirely successful outcome of the International Voice Symposium held in August 1987 was a great tonic. The idea that the Department of ENT surgery at Bangour should stage such an ambitious event was his alone. The initial planning was undertaken by him, supported by his wife, and a small group of staff.

The Symposium faculty included every world authority on the subject of voice reproduction including Professor Staffieri, the Italian founder of the famous Staffieri Technique, Professor Donald Shumrick from the USA, Professor P H Damste from Holland—the father of Oesophageal Speech— and Waryam Singh's good friend, the highly respected Professor M Hirano from Japan. At first accommodation at Bangour dictated that the number of delegates be limited to 250, but over 300 individuals applied from thirty-eight countries and overflow facilities had to be provided. The success of the Symposium placed the Ear, Nose and Throat department of Bangour General Hospital firmly on the world medical map. Following the Symposium, Waryam Singh has been in great demand to lecture and demonstrate his technique in many different parts of the world. At the same time, more and more patients from further and further afield have been referred to Bangour for his expert treatment. These patients include one of the world's richest men, but no matter who the patient, whether an Arab oil millionaire or a parish priest from Stirlingshire, Waryam Singh ensures that all receive the same skilled treatment and the chance to speak for themselves after surgery on their throat.

Ear, Nose and Throat surgery has made dramatic advances over the forty years it has been represented in West Lothian. With the use of new techniques and operating procedures, and by expanding their traditional surgical skills to include aspects of Plastic Surgery, General Surgery and Neurosurgery while working closely with colleagues in these fields, the repertoire of the Ear, Nose and Throat surgeon has increased considerably.

These developments have been supported by both the Scottish Home and Health Department and the Lothian Health Board who assisted in funding for a research laboratory.

SPEECH THERAPY

Speech Therapy as a profession began in the 1940s but it was 1949 before a part time speech therapist was employed to work in the Bangour Hospital, mainly with patients who had suffered from strokes. So far as the hospital records show Miss Edna Butfield was the only speech therapist ever to be employed directly by the Bangour Hospital Board of Management. Unfortunately Miss Butfield was not replaced when she left West Lothian in the mid 1950s. From then until 1974, speech therapy services for Bangour patients were provided on an *ad hoc* basis by the Public Health Department speech therapist at the request of the medical staff.

The 1974 re-organisation of the National Health Service made it possible for the Community Chief Speech Therapist to offer a limited, $1\frac{1}{2}$ days a week, service to Bangour General Hospital Medical and Ear, Nose and Throat Departments. As demand escalated and the scope of the speciality expanded, the speech therapy input from the Community Service to the hospital was increased to one full-time and one part-time therapist, who were employed to meet the demands of the hospital at the time of the move to phase one of St John's Hospital at Howden in 1989.

In recent years, developments have included the inception of a very active laryngectomy club, started in February 1984 at Bangour General Hospital. It is affiliated to the National Association of Laryngectomy Clubs, and its main function is as a support group for patients and their families/friends in the West Lothian area. Meetings are held monthly in the hospital and range from informal discussion to lectures or social events, one of the highlights being the annual dinner/dance. It provides an advisory service for patients about to undergo laryngectomy and has also donated equipment to the ENT Unit. Having initially been chaired by the Speech Therapist, it is now run entirely by the patients with support from the Speech Therapy Department.

There is close involvement with the ENT Department and the Voice Research Programme. In January 1988, the Speech Therapy Department became involved with the ENT Department in a major project for the analysis of alaryngeal speech. This was to look at the speech of neoglottis, oesophogeal and traceo-oesophogeal patients, and to compare this with that of a 'normal' control group. A number of interesting results have been obtained, in particular, it transpired that the speech of neoglottis speakers can be related very closely to that of 'normals'. Results have been obtained via a series of recordings carried out in the Voice Laboratory, which was set up after the successful International Voice Symposium 1987 conference. The project has just completed its first two year period, but it is hoped to extend this further.

As care of the elderly has increased in importance, developments in this area have included a service to the Bangour and Whitburn Day Hospitals, where patients have been treated in groups as well as individually. Recently it has been necessary to form a support group for dysphasia sufferers and their carers.

With the increasing range of patients treated by the Plastic and Facio-maxillary surgeons and in the Burns Unit, the expertise speech therapists have developed and are expanding is much in demand.

Children have not been seen by the therapists in Bangour General Hospital—most are referred and treated in the community. Consultants in Bangour General Hospital who have child patients at out-patient clinics refer to the community therapists as do those at the Royal Hospital for Sick Children in Edinburgh. The opening of a Paediatric Unit within St John's Hospital has allowed us to have a Paediatric Speech Therapist based there for five sessions a week.

Speech Therapists also make a major contribution to the West Lothian College of Nursing, lecturing to nursing students in their Medicine module, in their Communication with the Handicapped Child module and to nursing staff doing the Post Graduate Plastic Surgery course.

In every respect, from very low beginnings in 1949, the Speech Therapy Department has become an integral part of the life and work of Bangour General Hospital, liaising closely with the community it serves.

OPHTHALMOLOGY DEPARTMENT

The ophthalmology department was started in 1955. Before that date all West Lothian patients had to attend the Eye Department in the Royal Infirmary of Edinburgh for both out patient care or admission. The new department in West Lothian was housed in Wards Q7 and 8 at the north end of the surgical block. The wards were specially adapted to provide a small operating theatre with an adjacent anaesthetic room. There was a separate out patient clinic area with male and female wards at each end of the department. Children and adults were treated in the department for elective surgery such as cataract extractions, glaucoma operations, and for the correction of squints, retinal detachments and a wide range of emergency procedures also. The nursing staff had to be very versatile in those days and the ward sister was responsible for patient care in the wards, the operating theatre and the out patient clinic.

The first consultant appointed to the department was Dr T A S Boyd, who left for Edmonton, Alberta, and was succeeded in turn by Dr James Hughes and Dr N L Stokoe, both of whom moved to appointments in Edinburgh. They were followed by Dr Bill Haining who moved to Dundee University Medical School in 1968. Dr Haining was succeeded by the hospital's present consultant ophthalmologist, Dr Geoffrey Millar, whose father Tommy Millar had been one of the original general surgeons working in the Annexe of Bangour Village Hospital at its inception in 1940. The Millars lived in a house in Dechmont from 1940 until 1941 and little did Geoffrey ever expect to come back to West Lothian as a Consultant Ophthalmologist working in the hospital that his father had helped to found.

There has always been a very close relationship between the ophthalmology department in West Lothian and the Regional Service based in Edinburgh. Patients from Edinburgh occasionally came to West Lothian for their treatment to help shorten the Edinburgh waiting time for operations.

Dr Millar recalls an emergency operation one Saturday morning when the electric magnet broke down while it was being used to remove a metal fragment from an injured man's eye.

Help was summoned and the Lothians and Borders Police came to our rescue by transporting another magnet to Bangour from the Edinburgh Royal Infirmary at high speed to allow the operation to be successfully completed.

On another occasion, the repainting work in the ward had run beyond the anticipated time and patients were due to be admitted for operation. The only way in which this could be done was by asking the men and women patients to share the same ward with dividing screens between the sexes. All went well until one lady refused admission and complained to the South East of Scotland Regional Hospital Board who ordered us to stop what has subsequently become common practice in many hospitals. Yet another Bangour 'first' which was obviously well ahead of its time.

In 1975, after the Princess Alexandra Eye Pavilion of the Royal Infirmary was opened in Edinburgh, in patient surgical services for eye patients were transferred there and the accommodation in Wards Q7 and 8 was expanded and upgraded to allow the development of a specialist orthopaedic service. The Ophthalmology out patient clinic was moved to share facilities with Plastic Surgery in 'T' block, where it remained until the opening of St John's Hospital at Howden.

Unfortunately, the move to Edinburgh coincided with a considerable lengthening of the waiting list for eye operations as a result of the increasing numbers of older people in the population and the availability of a wide range of new techniques giving better vision after cataract operations. In addition operating time at the Princess Alexandra Eye Pavilion was limited and, in order to treat more patients and keep the waiting list under control, eye surgery was once again started at Bangour General Hospital in 1987. With the co-operation of the Gynaecology Department it was possible to operate once a fortnight and I was able to bring in up to five children who required surgery to correct their squints.

The major problem on the ophthalmology department waiting list was the vast number of elderly patients requiring the removal of a cataract and the implantation of new lenses which would allow these virtually blind old people to see once again. A series of 'cataract surgery blitzes' were undertaken over four weeks in 1988 and 1989 when the general surgical nursing staff in Ward Q4 and Q theatre turned their hands to the unfamiliar task of caring for older patients undergoing cataract extraction with lens implantation. One hundred and thirty-five operations were carried out with equipment bought or borrowed and the experienced help of a ward sister seconded from the Princess Alexandra Eye Pavilion to Bangour.

However [Dr Miller emphasized], the 'cataract surgery blitzes' would not have been possible without the mass of enthusiasm and good will from the many Bangour staff who participated and the very flexible and encouraging approach of the Hospital Management Group. In addition, the whole community of West Lothian played their part in these surgical 'blitzes' by raising over £9,000 through the good offices of the *Lothian Courier*. These funds were used to help defray the costs of these very delicate operations.

CARE OF THE ELDERLY

Dr Bill Conacher was Bangour General Hospital's first Consultant Physician specialising in the Care of the Elderly or 'Geriatrics'. The term 'Geriatrics' was coined in 1911 by a Jewish physician working in New York and he used it in the title of a textbook. In practical terms, the real pioneer was a female physician, Dr Marjory Warren, who developed a special medical unit for the care of the elderly in the West Middlesex Hospital, London, just before the Second World War. At this time in the United Kingdom, Care of the Elderly comprised of a few private nursing homes for the rich and poorhouses for the vast majority of frail elderly people. St Michael's Hospital, Linlithgow, which eventually came into partnership with Bangour General Hospital in 1982 was one of the latter types of hospital.

Shortly after the creation of the National Health Service in 1948, the medical society for the Care of the Elderly was established, but its members were mainly based in London. In Scotland, Professor Noah Morris in the Chair of Materia Medica at Glasgow University was very forward looking in this field and it was one of his junior colleagues. Dr O T Brown who became the first Consultant in Scotland to be appointed a specialist in Geriatric Medicine. Dr O T Brown was appointed in 1951 to work in Dundee and Dr Bill Conacher joined him at Maryfield Hospital as his first senior registrar in 1958.

> I was advised that Geriatric Medicine would be an expanding field of practice as a progressively larger proportion of the country's population would become elderly.

Accordingly Dr Conacher went to work in Dundee where he found Geriatrics a rewarding specialty. It proved to be the case that it was also an expanding specialty, for, after only fifteen months at Maryfield Hospital he was appointed Consultant Physician at Bangour General Hospital with responsibility for setting up a Geriatric Service in West Lothian. Dr Conacher started work in March 1960 and at that time the total population in West Lothian, which included Bo'ness and South Queensferry, was about 97,000 of whom approximately 10 per cent were age 65 or more. By 1989 the overall population of West Lothian, excluding Bo'ness and South Queensferry had increased, mainly due to the new town of Livingston, to approximately 145,000 of whom approximately 6,000 people are aged over 75. It is predicted that this number will increase by 23 per cent before the end of this century so the Care of the Elderly continues to be an expanding specialty in medicine.

One of Dr Conacher's priorities when he took up his post in 1960 was to re-design and upgrade two derelict wards (P7 and P8) in the medical block as an active geriatric assessment and rehabilitation unit for elderly, physically frail patients. This included providing improved access to toilet facilities and trying to persuade the administration to produce significantly higher levels of nursing care.

In 1960 West Lothian was blessed with four small hospitals providing care in the community and Dr Conacher managed to incorporate these hospitals into the overall geriatric service by the simple technique of unifying their medical record systems and visiting them on a regular basis. These hospitals proved a very valuable resource because it allowed the elderly patients to be located reasonably near to their family. St Michael's Hospital at Linlithgow was built as a Poorhouse in 1850 and the original building was still occupied in 1960, mainly by the 'indigent poor' although there were also forty beds in a less ancient hospital block, which more recently has been replaced by a purpose built modern unit of thirty-two beds. Drumshoreland Hospital, built in 1888, was originally a fever hospital for Mid Lothian before it became a Geriatric Long Stay Hospital. Drumshoreland Hospital was eventually closed in the spring of 1990 having served the community for 102 years, the remaining patients in the hospital being transferred to the Geriatric Unit in 'P' block in Bangour General Hospital. Tippethill Hospital, a fever hospital built at the turn of the century to serve Linlithgowshire, looked after a mixture of patients under the care of local General Practitioners until it became a full time Long Stay Geriatric Hospital. The fourth small hospital in this group was Bo'ness Hospital. Between 1960 and 1973 this hospital was looked after by West Lothian but in 1973 it was officially transferred to the care of the Forth Valley Health Board. It was not until the mid 1980s, however, that full medical responsibility for all patients, out patient clinics, physiotherapy service and X-Ray department was finally taken over.

In addition to the development of an integrated Bangour General Hospital and Community Hospital service for geriatric patients, Dr Conacher also championed the cause of the establishment of Day Hospitals where elderly patients could come to meet friends and have their general health and welfare reviewed by the very caring staff, many of whom have worked in the Bangour Day Hospital since its opening in 1981 in the former Tuberculosis Isolation Ward—'R9'. A second purpose built day hospital was opened in the Whitburn Health Centre in 1985. There is also a voluntary day care centre working in conjunction with St Michael's Hospital in Linlithgow as a result of local community fund raising efforts and this service started in 1987.

Dr Conacher is the first to admit that these major achievements, with regard to the provision of an integrated hospital in patient and day hospital service in West Lothian, could not have been achieved without tremendous support and encouragement from nursing and medical colleagues.

In particular I would single out Dr Graham Buckley and Dr Bob Finnie who have, over the last fifteen years, worked as hospital practitioners in the geriatric service in West Lothian, in addition to carrying out their duties as General Practitioners in Livingston. Their presence in the geriatric service has helped promote a good rapport between hospital and general practice. We've also managed to develop a good rapport between the geriatric service and the many other hospital departments with which we need close links and this particularly applies to Dr Charles Corser and his colleagues in the Psychogeriatric Unit at Bangour Village Hospital.

More recently, a particularly valuable and close co-operation has been developed between the hospital and the West Lothian Social Work department with its six homes for the care of the physically frail and elderly and nowadays it is possible to aim at ensuring that the most appropriate type of care is given to each individual patient, whether in a West Lothian District Home for the Elderly, in the Day Hospital or a Long Stay Hospital Bed.

Shortly before Dr Conacher's retiral in February 1989 the West Lothian Geriatric Service was visited by the Scottish Hospital Advisory Service. This committee carried out a detailed analysis of West Lothian's Geriatric Service between 5 and 9 December and on 21 December 1988. The conclusion of the report is worth quoting.

If there is little that is critical in this report it is because there is little to criticise. Those who have established the service have considerable cause for satisfaction and we have every confidence in those respon-sible for its continued development.

Signed Dr A Drummond, Director.

This report is praise indeed following detailed scrutiny of a service which started from nothing in 1960. Dr Conacher has handed over the Care of the Elderly in West Lothian to Dr John Wilson who was appointed as Consultant Geriatrician to West Lothian in October 1988 after spending some of his training in general medicine in Geriatrics in Bangour General Hospital. Early in 1990 Dr Wilson was joined by Dr D L Farquhar. Care of the Elderly will take up increasing proportions of medical resources and the service that has been established in West Lothian as it moves into Phase II of St John's Hospital at Howden towards the end of the twentieth century is well set to face the many challenges lying ahead.

ANAESTHETIC SERVICES

Sir James Young Simpson, the discoverer of the anaesthetic properties of Chloroform, was born in Bathgate on 7 June 1811, the son of a baker. Following his final examinations in medicine, he became a member of the Royal College of Surgeons in 1830 while only 19 years old. He then devoted himself to a career in Obstetrics and became increasingly concerned at the pain which surgery and childbirth produced.

Chloroform was discovered in 1831 but it wasn't until the 4 November 1847 that Dr Simpson, at the suggestion of a Mr David Waldie of Linlithgow, obtained a sample of the substance from the Edinburgh firm of Duncan & Flockhart. At the end of a family supper party that night, Dr Simpson and his friends carried out a series of experiments which resulted in the drug being used for the very first time as an anaesthetic agent on 15 November 1847 in the Royal Infirmary of Edinburgh.

After many early objections, anaesthesia developed as a speciality in its own right and at the setting up of Bangour General Hospital during the Second World War all Anaesthetic Services were provided initially by the Neurosurgical Anaesthetists, under Dr Alan Brown, who were working with Professor Norman Dott in the Neurosurgical Unit of Bangour Village Hospital prior to that unit moving into Edinburgh. Dr Brown was ably assisted by a number of lady anaesthetists covering a variety of anaesthetic sessions for the duration of the war and the early post war years.

In 1952 Dr Hugh Boyd was appointed as the first full-time Consultant Anaesthetist in Bangour. At that time he was assisted by two experienced Senior Hospital Medical Officers, Dr Teddy Norman and Dr Nancy Muir, with one rotating Senior Registrar from the Royal Infirmary and one junior anaesthetist in training. Dr Boyd was a bachelor who lived in the hospital and was regularly found in the wards at all times of the day and night. In fact Bangour General Hospital was his main interest in life, the other being photography. His photographs of the home of Sir James Young Simpson in Bathgate, prior to its demolition, have been gratefully accepted by historians of anaesthesia for safe keeping. Dr Boyd's proudest achievement in anaesthesia was when he was able to procure for Bangour General Hospital the first patient ventilator in the South East of Scotland.

The staffing levels in the Anaesthetic Department remained the same until 1964 when Dr Norman moved to a Consultant post in South Lothian. Dr Henry Turner was then appointed as the second full-time Consultant Anaesthetist in Bangour. During the period between Dr Turner accepting his appointment and actually taking up his post, Dr Nancy Muir died of renal failure and Dr Boyd, while on a holiday cruise out of Southampton, suffered a stroke which resulted in Dr Turner arriving at Bangour as the 'Consultant in Charge' with no colleagues! Dr Boyd recovered partially from his stroke but was unable to continue practising Anaesthesia. He did, however, continue to live in the hospital keeping up his old contacts and enjoying a coffee with his colleagues for a number of years before he finally retired to become the first resident to enter Strathbrock Home in Broxburn— a fact of which he was very proud!

The Anaesthetic Department functioned for the next eighteen months with Dr Turner assisted by a series of locum appointments. This was rectified by the appointment in late 1965 of Dr Connie Howie and then, during the following year, Dr Alan Grace, both of whom had been junior anaesthetists in Bangour during their training. Dr Howie and Dr Grace were particularly involved with the Plastic Surgeons and the planning and commissioning of the Regional Specialist Burns Unit servicing the whole of the South East of Scotland as well as part of the Highlands. This Unit was officially opened on the 25 June 1968, by the Very Rev R Leonard Small, an ex-moderator of the Church of Scotland who started his ministry in the 1930s in St John's Church in Bathgate and who is father of one of the present Consultant Anaesthetists working in Bangour. The work load of the Burns Unit has steadily increased over the years with the problems of smoke inhalation from the fumes produced by foam filled furniture in house fires. These fumes result in severe respiratory injuries which aggravate the burns to such an extent that many of the patients require life support and artificial ventilation for long periods of time, placing great demands on the Anaesthetic Staff.

The advances made by the Anaesthetic Department in Bangour over and above the simple number of anaesthetics given, i.e. 5,000 per year in 1960 to 14,000 per year in 1989, have been in various fields. A number of anaesthetic agents have disappeared from our practice including Chloroform, Ethyl Chloride, Cyclopropane and most recently Trichloroethylene or Trilene which can be smelt in every dry cleaning shop in the country as it is the basis for cleaning agents for the removal of grease from clothing.

Safety in Anaesthesia has always been a primary consideration and very high standards have been achieved, the death rate being in the region of one per 10,000 anaesthetics given. The second consideration has always been the relief of pain, the primary motivating force which led Sir James Young Simpson to the discovery of Chloroform. Post operative pain and the pain in childbirth still remain important considerations for a patient. Over the past seven years Anaesthetists have introduced a technique of giving pain relief by infusing powerful opiate drugs like morphine directly into a patient's veins. This technique requires the drug to be injected in a controlled manner by a specially designed syringe driver pump. When this technique was started in Bangour there were only two syringe pumps so this sophisticated type of pain relief could only be offered to two patients at any one time. In 1986 Theatre Staff—enthusiastically misled by the Operating Department Attendant George Kerr—organised a sponsored parachute jump in the North of England as part of a fund raising activity. This resulted in a lot of hair raising and bone shaking escapades but produced the sum of £3,000 which, in conjunction with the generous support of the staff of Levi Jeans factory in Whitburn who had guaranteed £3 for every £1 raised by the staff, resulted in the magnificent sum of £12,000 being donated. This money purchased a further six syringe pumps for pain relief as well as other specialised instruments for the Department of Surgery. At a reception in the hospital the Union Representatives from Levi's and the Theatre Staff were shown the equipment provided by their fund raising activities. Approximately some six months later one of the Levi representatives who had been at that reception had to have an operation and benefited from the pain relief provided by one of the pumps which she and her colleagues at Levi's had helped fund—a fine example of a community benefiting from its own fund raising efforts on behalf of its own hospital. Incidentally, nowadays such fund raising activities as parachute jumping by untrained personnel are not encouraged as it tends to cost the National Health Service more to patch up the casualties than is raised by the activity!

Pain relief in childbirth is another area in which the Bangour Anaesthetic Department has been able to make considerable advances in the 1980s. The provision of an Epidural Service to women in labour has expanded over the years from approximately forty per annum in 1976, for purely medical indications, to around 360 per year in 1989. Provision of an Epidural Service is very demanding on Anaesthetic manpower and only when the number of new babies born in a hospital is over 2,500 per year is it possible to employ the extra manpower which would allow us to provide every woman who wants an Epidural during their labour with this facility. At the moment the number of new babies born at Bangour remains approximately 1,800 each year with the result that the Anaesthetic Department is not able to employ enough staff to offer a full Epidural Service. However, every effort is made to comply with the patients' wishes but this is not always possible and will prove to be a particularly difficult problem over the years of split site working between Bangour General Hospital and St John's Hospital at Howden. In the 1980s pain relief provided for women by Epidural Anaesthetics in labour has been adapted in such a way that patients having major abdominal surgery and lower limb surgery can have their post operative pain relieved. A special catheter is inserted into the spinal column at the beginning of an operation and a constant infusion of a weak local anaesthetic combined with a powerful pain relieving drug—Heroin—is started prior to the patient waking up at the end of their operation. This mixture of substances provides almost total pain relief for the following two days while the infusion is continued through the Epidural Catheter. Looking after any patient who is receiving any form of Epidural Anaesthetic places a major strain on Anaesthetic and Nursing Staff because of the very close supervision they must be given but these types of Anaesthetics have proved to be a major advance in the relief of pain in childbirth and after operations.

The Anaesthetic Department has also had to respond to developments in surgical practice. The modern technique of using an Operating Microscope in conjunction with the development of Micro Vascular Surgery, where free flaps of skin, fat and muscle can be transplanted to cover deformities or defects, or where fingers or limbs accidentally amputated in the course of work or play, can be sewn back on, have led to major problems for Anaesthetists.

A recent case where a patient had four fingers amputated by a chain saw illustrates the problem: the operation started at 8.00 p.m. and finished at 2.00 p.m. the following day—a total of eighteen hours for one case!—a trying time for everyone concerned, the surgeon, the anaesthetist, nurses but, most important of all, the patient.

Other developing areas of interest affecting the Anaesthetic Service is the intensive care of the severely ill or injured patient. This specialty is very demanding on highly skilled and trained medical and nursing personnel and requires the most expensive modern equipment. A start was made in the development of Intensive Care facilities in Bangour Hospital in the side room of one of the Surgical Wards in the early 1980s, as well as in the Plastic Surgery and Burns Unit. A suitably planned Intensive Care Unit will be provided when St John's Hospital at Howden is opened in 1992.

Dr Colin Small has been instrumental in developing a team of staff including some of his fellow anaesthetists and the Pharmacy Department to run a Total Parenteral Nutritional Service for severely ill or injured patients. This service requires the placing of a delicate feeding catheter into the main vein of the right side of the heart and thereafter the patient receives a balanced diet, at a cost of approximately £77 per day, by direct injection into the bloodstream.

As the demands on the Anaesthetic Department have increased over the years so have the number of staff, and the one-man band initiated by Dr Hugh Boyd in 1952 has expanded to a team of seven Consultants, one Hospital Practitioner, Dr John Donald from Howden Health Centre, Livingston, and six junior staff including a rotating senior registrar coming out from Edinburgh.

Bangour Hospital may not have had all the requirements in the term of facilities and equipment expected of a modern hospital, such as will be provided in St John's Hospital at Howden, but it always had a very special atmosphere which made it a pleasant place in which to be a patient, and the staff, many of whom have worked there all their professional life, will always remember it with affection.

Chapter Eleven

Meanwhile Back at the Village

While the physical structure of Bangour Village Hospital may have changed little since the war, the work going on within has altered steadily over the years. Developments have come about, firstly as a result of changing trends in psychiatric practice nationwide and, secondly, due to reorganisation within the local Health Service. These influences have acted together to link 'Old Bangour' even more closely with the community of West Lothian, to their mutual benefit.

It was not until the mid 1950s that the Village Hospital first admitted patients from West Lothian, their psychiatric care having previously been the responsibility of Hartwood and Bellsdyke Hospitals. In 1956 Bangour ceased to function as the pauper lunatic asylum for the City of Edinburgh, although it was not until 1974 that it stopped admitting patients from Edinburgh and accepted West Lothian as its sole catchment area.

Between these dates very much more effective drug treatments for the major psychoses or mental illnesses were introduced into psychiatric practice. This allowed for less emphasis to be placed on custody in caring for the mentally ill with the result that considerably fewer patients have been required to spend prolonged periods, often years, in the wards of the hospital. It was Doctor, later Professor, Kenneth Macrae, the Physician Superintendent at the hospital between 1957 and 1969, who is credited with having opened the doors of the locked wards at Bangour and the philosophy persists today of encouraging patients to utilise the space and tranquillity offered by the grounds of the hospital.

The improved treatments also mean that many patients have been rehabilitated from the hospital back into the community and that ever increasing numbers have had contact with the psychiatric services without ever entering the hospital grounds. While Bangour Village Hospital remained responsible for patients from North Edinburgh, out patient clinics were established at the Western General Hospital, the Northern General Hospital, Eastern General Hospital, Bo'ness Hospital, Leith Hospital and most significantly, at Sighthill Health Centre.

Sighthill Health Centre was one of the first purpose-built health centres

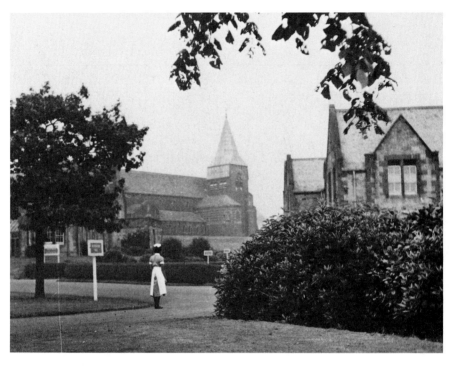

Fig. 56   The War Memorial Church catches the attention of a nurse going on duty.

to be opened in the United Kingdom, where groups of family doctors saw their patients. The health centre also provided treatment facilities for health visitors, district nurses and some specialist clinics. Dr Betty Magill, one of the consultants at Bangour, established an out patient clinic at Sighthill in 1959, the first such clinic to be opened in the United Kingdom. General practice based psychiatric clinics are only now being widely recognised as the most appropriate way of treating patients suffering from minor psychiatric disorders but there are few, if any, areas which have developed such a service as successfully as West Lothian. Clinics are now held in Armadale, Bathgate, Blackburn, Linlithgow, Whitburn, Craigshill and Howden Health Centres, Livingston and Broxburn. Few people in West Lothian have to travel to Old Bangour for psychiatric help should they choose not to do so.

The link between the hospital service and general practitioners is one of the strongest features of the medical service in West Lothian. Within psychiatry the contact has not been restricted to the development of out patient clinics. Psychiatric nurses have worked from health centres seeing patients either at the request of the general practitioner or the psychiatrist. Such community psychiatric nurses work alongside health visitors, domiciliary

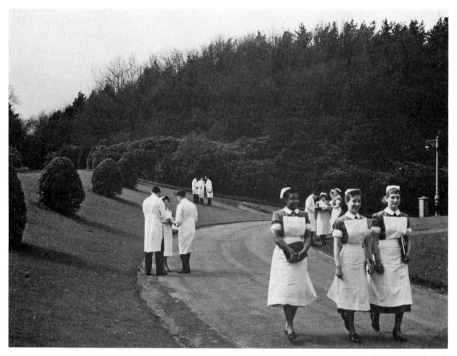

Fig. 57 Student nurses strolling between classes through the beautiful grounds of the Village in 1958. The nurse on the left was from Barbados.

midwives and district nurses, helping to fuse together the teamwork necessary in the care of those with psychiatric problems.

Providing out-patient and domiciliary care within the community is of benefit to large numbers of patients. Approximately 8,000 psychiatric clinic appointments are filled each year in West Lothian and of these 1,500 are taken up by out patients attending for the first time. However, there remains those for whom more is required. Some will always have to be admitted to hospital but the provision of day hospital facilities can help to minimise the number. Further extensions of the provision of community based psychiatric care in West Lothian are planned and the development of an acute day hospital has been accorded the highest priority by the Hospital Management Team. Such a facility would further decrease the need for patients with psychiatric problems to enter hospital and minimise the time spent in hospital by those who are admitted.

What of the unfortunate patients who were admitted to hospital in large numbers prior to the development of effective treatments and whose often prolonged stay has institutionalised them, making them totally dependent on the hospital? The problems which prevented such people leaving hospital were largely social, with lack of housing, unemployment and deficient self-care skills paramount. The return to the community or rehabilitation of long-term psychiatric patients has been ubiquitous and thanks to the good links within West Lothian, Bangour Village Hospital has been particularly successful. There are many individual examples of this success but perhaps the single most telling statistic is the fall in the hospital patient population from its peak of 1,200 to the present level of just over 500. Much of the credit for this must be accorded to Dr Alistair McKechnie who only ceased to be Physician Superintendent in 1989 when he was seconded to the Mental Welfare Commission. It is also noteworthy that in 1987 Dr Ollie Wilson, a Consultant at Bangour from 1977 to 1989, was elected President of the World Association for Psychosocial Rehabilitation.

The first requirement to be met in order to facilitate the exodus of patients was housing. In the early 1970s the hospital approached Livingston Development Corporation who responded magnificently by offering complete blocks of flats. However, it was decided that this might only serve to create psychiatric ghettoes within the community and instead houses in Don Drive, Victoria Street and Hobart Street in the Craigshill district and one further house in the Deans area of Livingston were accepted. These provided successful homes for groups of former hospital patients for a number of years, but with the earlier occupants moving on to independent living or returning to the hospital due to increasing age and infirmity. The house in Deans is the only Group Home remaining in the Livingston area.

Following negotiations with the West Lothian District Council a further two houses have been acquired in the Bathgate area and these are currently very successful Group Homes.

In more recent years it has been recognised that there are those with psychiatric problems who will always have difficulty in living independently outwith hospital but who may do so with ongoing assistance. To provide for such people, a range of supported accommodation has been developed in conjunction with voluntary bodies, in particular the Scottish Association for Mental Health and Penumbra. These projects have allowed in excess of thirty-five previously long-term psychiatric patients to return to the community without any fear that their quality of life may suffer in the process.

So successful have these ventures been that it is hard to recall the initial anxieties expressed by representatives of the communities where the accommodation was to be sited. The concept of 'not in my back yard' is not restricted to the affluent areas of major cities, where it is all too prevalent; it has also had to be tackled in West Lothian. However, thanks to good communication and down-to-earth commonsense it has not proved insurmountable. It has been of considerable help that, often, members of the hospital staff who have known the patients for many years are themselves potential neighbours. Many difficult meetings were defused by Nursing Officer Andy Ashcroft announcing with confidence that he, his wife and their young children would be living practically next door to one group home and that this caused him no concern.

The housing need for former hospital patients has thus been met very successfully in West Lothian. What of the accompanying problems of occupation and day-to-day living? These have been and are continuing to be met by the West Lothian Day Hospital based on the Village Hospital campus and three offshoots in Whitburn, Livingston and Bathgate. The Day Hospital itself provides post-discharge follow-up treatment and occupational therapy for fifty former patients on a sessional basis, with staff also providing support for individuals within their own homes where necessary. The '81 Club, the name of which derives from its year of origin, was developed by Dr Joan Thomson to provide a community based resource in Whitburn and, since 1987, a similar provision has existed in Bathgate. These facilities are the result of collaboration between the hospital, Whitburn Community Centre, and the West Lothian College of Further Education in Bathgate and have proved very successful. Perhaps even more exciting has been the development of a club in Deans Community High School in conjunction with the Community Education Department. This unique alliance between psychiatry and education has proved not only an outstanding success for those who attend, but has also allowed hospital staff to work with teachers and pupils from the school, considerably lessening the stigma of mental illness in the process.

The three community based centres provide places for over one hundred attenders who are able to take part in a wide range of social and therapeutic activities including keep fit, drama, cooking and photography.

It is entirely appropriate that the history of Bangour Village Hospital since the war should concentrate on community developments but, within the hospital, change has been considerable. An increasing awareness of the differing needs of separate groups of the mentally ill has led to a specialisation of services. The needs of the young have resulted in the development of the Adolescent Unit, described elsewhere, and at the other end of the age spectrum, the early 1970s saw plans for a comprehensive service for the elderly with mental disorder at Bangour Village Hospital, using the pioneering work of Dr R A Robinson at the Crichton Royal Hospital in Dumfries as a model. When Dr Robinson moved to Lothian he took responsibility for the service pertaining to North Edinburgh, which eventually moving from its base at Bangour to the purpose-built Royal Victoria Hospital.

The West Lothian service was initially in the hands of Dr Donald Beattie but since 1974 the driving force behind its development has been Dr Charles Corser. Under his guidance and with the enthusiastic support of two charge nurses, Sister Betty Brown and Mr Bob Ross, Ward 32 at the hospital has become a very active psychogeriatric unit providing assessment, treatment

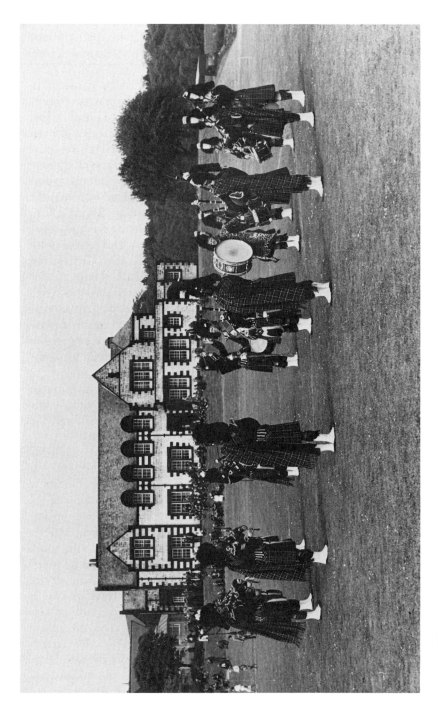

Fig. 58 Fund-raising and liaison with the community have always been an integral part of life at the Village with the annual fete being a major event in the fund-raising calendar.

and respite facilities. The importance of supporting the main carers of the elderly, that is the families, was noted at an early stage and day hospital places were provided in 1977 using a wooden building vacated by the School of Nursing. This 'temporary' day hospital functioned for over twelve years eventually being replaced by the Parkview Day Unit on the hospital campus.

As with all aspects of the psychiatric service in West Lothian, there was an early commitment to community care. This initially depended on the goodwill of the ward-based nursing staff but within the past five years the appointment of two community psychiatric nurses specifically for the elderly has allowed many more people to be cared for within their own homes. Equally important has been the close liaison with the other statutory and voluntary bodies responsible for the elderly, a feature which will be increasingly important in the years ahead.

Specialisation has also occurred in the areas of forensic psychiatry, to provide for those whose psychiatric difficulties lead them to transgress society's rules of accepted behaviour and further developments are planned to combat the problems of substance abuse with the associated risk of HIV infection. A close relationship has always existed between Bangour Village Hospital and its annexe, and with an ever-expanding liaison service the links between psychiatrists in West Lothian and their colleagues in other branches of hospital medicine will certainly live on, following the move to St John's.

The integration of Bangour Village Hospital with West Lothian has been further enhanced by the Livingston Experiment. The general impact of this has been described elsewhere and it has been no less influential on the psychiatric service. Dr John Henderson who, after a spell as Physician Superintendent between 1969 and 1972, moved to work with the World Health Organisation, was very involved in the planning but it was the late Dr John Rae who largely oversaw the implementation.

It is often said that psychiatry and general practice have much in common and this was certainly confirmed by the initial incumbents of the posts split between Livingston Health Centres and Bangour Village Hospital, four of whom became full-time psychiatrists. Of these four, Dr Corser and Dr Jim McMichael remain on the Village Hospital staff. The present postholders, Dr John Ferguson, Dr Ian Buchan and Dr Nawal Bagaria, whilst perhaps not planning to move into psychiatry full time, contribute very significantly to the service and act as a permanent reminder of where the vast majority of patients with psychiatric disorders are treated—in the GPs' surgery.

PSYCHOLOGY AT BANGOUR HOSPITALS 1940–1990

In 1990, the Village Hospital commemorated fifty years since the first appointment of a psychologist to work at Bangour. This is a long history for what is a relatively new profession.

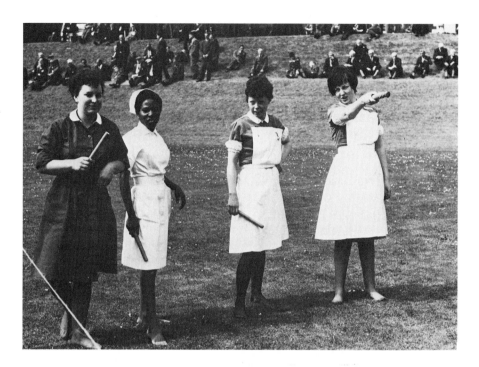

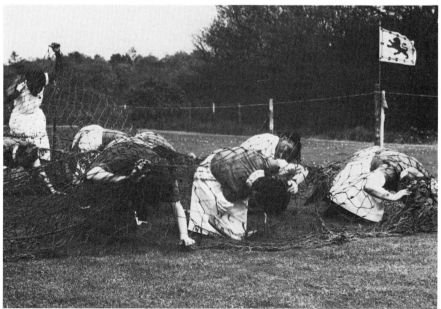

Figs. 59 and 60   A highly competitive group of nurses enjoying the fete.

THE 1940s

Bangour General Hospital was extensively used during the First World War and preparations for its use for the expected casualties in the Second World War were made before hostilities began. These included the use of Wards 9 and 32 at Bangour Village Hospital by the Brain Injuries Unit for cases transferred from the Royal Infirmary of Edinburgh. A psychologist, Oliver Zangwill, was appointed as Rockefeller Research Scholar and worked as part of the Brain Injury Team in Edinburgh and at Bangour from 1940 to 1945.

Zangwill was concerned with some of the problems of rehabilitation faced by soldiers who suffered gunshot wounds to the head. His early papers, based on work done at Bangour, show that he adopted a scientific approach to neuropsychology and became regarded in international circles as one of the founders of the discipline of Neuropsychology. After leaving Bangour he returned to an academic career and in 1952 was appointed to the Chair of Psychology at Cambridge University. He later launched *Neuropsychologia*, a journal dedicated to neuropsychology, which he edited for some twenty years. Although an experimentalist himself he remained keen to see the results of laboratory investigations applied, where appropriate, in hospital settings. He was elected a Fellow of the Royal Society of London in 1977 and was President of the British Psychological Society in 1974–5.

By the time Zangwill left the Brain Injury Unit in Edinburgh and Bangour, the value of the clinical as well as the research role of the psychologist in the unit was established and arrangements were made with Professor Drever of the Psychology department at Edinburgh University to obtain the services of a lecturer, Miss Agnes Sladden, on a part-time basis. This proved particularly valuable and allowed the Psychology Department to collaborate in rehabilitation with the Speech and Occupational Therapy departments and with the Disablement Resettlement Officer who regularly attended discharge meetings.

With the resignation of Miss Sladden in 1949 the post continued with the appointment of Dr Jim Naughton, a graduate in Medicine and Psychology, who continued to provide a service at Bangour until the transfer of the services to the newly-built unit in the Western General Hospital in May 1960. The Brain Injury Unit had been renamed the Department of Surgical Neurology following its assimilation into the National Health Service when this was established. Dr Naughton comments that the transfer from Bangour to the Western General was 'not without regret for the loss of the amenity and fresh country air at Bangour'.

THE 1960s

There is a dearth of information about psychology at Bangour in the early 1960s and it is likely that there were no posts at that time. In 1960, however, both Edinburgh and Glasgow Universities started two-year post-graduate training courses for clinical psychologists, and psychology services in psychiatric hospitals began to be established as trained clinical psychologists became available.

At Bangour Village Hospital the first Basic Grade psychologist was Mr (now Dr) Gerry Greene who is now joint course organiser of the Glasgow University Clinical Psychology training course. At that time, in line with current practice, his main role was in carrying out psychometric assessments on adults and adolescents, as well as working in the alcohol unit where he was involved in some research. Teaching nurses on psychiatric nurse training courses at the College of Nursing at Bangour General Hospital was also an important aspect of his job.

The post became vacant in 1965 and the next incumbent was Mrs Mala Kapur who maintained the clinical, research and teaching roles already developed.

THE 1970s

In 1969 Mrs Kapur was joined by Mr David McIver who remained at Bangour Village Hospital until 1972 when he was appointed to a senior post at the Royal Edinburgh Hospital. Mrs Kapur left during 1970 and at that time a case was made by Mr McIver for the establishment of a Department of Clinical Psychology, headed by a principal psychologist with a number of junior staff covering different aspects of the clinical work within the hospital. The Board of Management accepted this argument and a principal grade post was established. Dr Alistair Philip was appointed to this head of department post in 1971 and under his direction the department grew from two posts to seven by 1975. These included Dr Felicity Buckley, Mr Alan Coupar, Dr Graham McColl, Ms Ann Green and Ms Fiona Cathcart. At all times the emphasis was on maintaining a balance between clinical work, research and teaching.

Dr McColl had particular expertise in Gestalt Therapy and ran a number of groups for staff as an aid to team development.

During the same period, Alistair Philip and Ann Green, were instrumental in creating a token economy system based in Ward 26. This was useful in developing skills in those patients who had been in Bangour Village Hospital for many years. However, after a time the appropriate facilities for maintaining these skills were no longer available in the long-stay area of Bangour Village Hospital or in the community. Nevertheless, many patients did benefit from the scheme, and the opportunities which it gave for nursing staff and psychologists to work closely and collaboratively together had lasting benefits.

In 1973 a post was established to provide a clinical psychology service in

Craigshill Health Centre in Livingston. Initially it was part of the Livingston Health Services Experiment, but when the Livingston Experiment officially came to an end the psychology post formally became part of the Bangour Village Hospital establishment. This post was filled by Miss Terry McAllister (later Griffiths) and was the first establishment of a full-time post in primary care in Britain. It was thanks to the forward thinking of Dr John Henderson (then Physician Superintendent), Dr Alistair Philip and the Health Services Experiment Team that the post was established.

During the 1970s the expansion of the department within Bangour Village Hospital ensured that both admission wards—child and adolescent service and psychogeriatric service—as well as the long-stay area, received psychological input.

THE 1980s

Dr Philip left Bangour Village Hospital in 1980 and Mrs Terry Griffiths then took over as head of department.

During the 1980s the emphasis has been on developing a comprehensive service throughout West Lothian, while continuing research and teaching commitments. Psychology services are provided to the psychiatric teams in the admission units at Bangour Village Hospital and to the Psychogeriatric, Rehabilitation, Child Psychiatry and Intensive Psychiatric Care Unit Teams. Also, during the 1980s there had been increased demand from Bangour General Hospital and, when required, services were provided to the Geriatric, Medical, and Burns and Plastic Surgery units.

Links with the community are strong, particularly through the rehabilitation team and the work undertaken in primary care which, since the end of the Livingston Experiment, has been assimilated into the work of the department and spread much more widely throughout West Lothian. Each psychologist has responsibility for designated Health Centres and is expected to develop a close working relationship with staff as well as dealing with referrals from the practice. Behavioural, cognitive and psychotherapeutic approaches are used with individuals and with groups. There is close collaboration with colleagues in medicine, nursing, occupational therapy and physiotherapy and inter-referral and shared care are frequent. As well as a wide range of clinical services, research and teaching remain important features of the department's workload.

Many clinical and teaching projects are undertaken each year. Recent examples are running 'Quality of Life' workshops for long-term care of psychogeriatric wards (Janice Whittick); teaching and case discussion with staff of Barnardos Day Care Centre (Artemis Curran); a Consumer Survey of Community Rehabilitation Services (Neil Rothwell).

The department's publication list continues to grow steadily and research

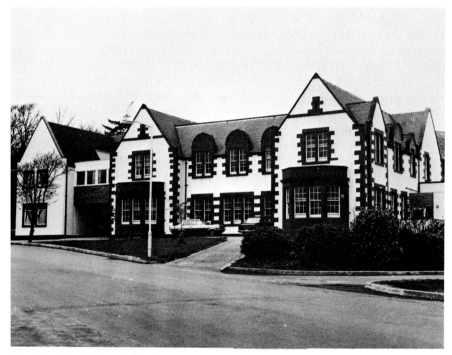

Fig. 61   The fabric of the villas in the Village requires constant upkeep to maintain
the high standard of finish as demonstrated in this photograph of Ward 7 in 1980.
The Works Department have a challenging role maintaining the Village and General
Hospitals at Bangour while developing St John's.

funds, particularly for work with the elderly, have been awarded by the
Scottish Home and Health Department to Ms Whittick.

THE 1990s

The changes in the tasks undertaken by clinical psychologists at Bangour
Village Hospital over the last fifty years have been indicative of changes in
the development of the profession as a whole. However, at Bangour we have
frequently been at the vanguard in translating these changes in thinking into
action. Only with the support of, and in collaboration with, other professions
working in West Lothian have these innovations been possible. We look
forward to the continuation of the psychology service and its development
to meet the challenge of the 1990s.

Chapter Twelve

The Enablers

The longest serving member of staff in the physiotherapy department at Bangour General Hospital is Mrs Margaret Sneddon, previously Margaret Hadfield, who came to Scotland for the first time in November 1955.

I am looking back over 35 years to try and remember my first impressions of Bangour. Two of us, newly qualified physiotherapists, arrived by train at Waverley Station, Edinburgh and stepped onto Scottish soil for the very first time in our lives in November 1955. We made our way to St Andrew's Square and climbed aboard a bus heading for Glasgow, asking the conductress to tell us when we had reached Bangour Hospital. When the bus passed the Broxburn sign, Bangour's postal address, we waited to be told that the next stop would be ours but no call came and soon we passed into Uphall, so we checked with the conductress and she was able to reassure us that we hadn't missed our destination. We were very tired and had large suitcases, coats over our arms and portable radios (much bigger than the present day pocket sized ones) and the thought of having to change buses appalled us. We finally alighted at Bangour Hospital gate. We had been told that there would be a bus to meet us but there was no sign of one. While waiting its arrival we were approached by a respectable looking gentleman who asked us where we had come from. When we told him he advised us strongly to return there straight away—'It isn't safe at Bangour, you need to sleep with a gun under your pillow'. All this happened in the inky darkness of a West Lothian night. We did not know anything about the Village Hospital. We had not even been up for an interview prior to being offered the job as, at that time, there were far more posts available than qualified physiotherapists to fill them. Accordingly we had been accepted on completion of application forms. Our next encounter was with the driver of a small van who said that he was a hospital engineer and that he would take our luggage to the nurses' home, where we were to be resident. We gladly let him take our cases but then wondered if we would ever see them again—and of course we did.

There were seven resident physiotherapists including the two of us. There was some class distinction as there were two separate dining rooms. The physiotherapists were included in the 'upper class' and dined with the sisters. We had our own sitting room with a radio which rarely worked. A coal fire was laid for us every day but it was very difficult to light and we ended up using most of our week's sugar ration trying to encourage the flames. All residents received weekly sugar and butter rations, a bag of biscuits and some fresh fruit. On your day off, breakfast in bed was a treat. You just put your room number on a slate the previous evening and it was nice to be woken by one of the maids with a tray the next morning.

The nurses' home was locked at 11 p.m. If you were out any later you had to contact the night sister who would send one of the male nurses to open up. There were wooden blocks inserted in the windows of the ground floor of the building to prevent them from opening more than 4 inches. Men were not allowed into the female staff room, not even husbands.

At this point it is worth appreciating that Margaret Hadfield was single when she came to work in the Bangour Hospitals having only just completed her physiotherapy training. Scotland obviously made a very favourable impression upon her because shortly after her arrival she met her husband to be, John Sneddon, who was one of the few male nurses living in the Bangour Village Hospital nurses' home, while undertaking his psychiatric nurse training. Margaret and John obviously managed to overcome the various rules and regulations segregating the 'upper class' qualified physiotherapist from the male psychiatric student nurse because they rapidly got to know each other well, fell in love and were married in Bathgate High Church in 1956.

John Sneddon successfully completed his psychiatric nurse training and graduated as the first man to win a gold medal in psychiatric nurse training in the United Kingdom. He was presented with his medal by Lord and Lady Roseberry, 48 hours after Margaret had presented him with his new-born daughter, Elizabeth. John Sneddon subsequently devoted his working life to the psychiatric services in West Lothian while Margaret devoted her professional skills to the physiotherapy patients in the hospital and community in West Lothian.

Mrs Sneddon continues:

The physiotherapy department in 1955 was in Bangour Village Hospital in the present occupational therapy department. The full staff compliment was ten physiotherapists and one remedial gymnast. We worked Monday to Friday and alternate Saturday mornings. There was no evening or Sunday cover. Miss Kathleen Prior was the Superintendent but she left during that year to be succeeded early in 1956 by Miss Letty Morrison. The department was quite large and contained several rooms of varying sizes. The main large treatment room was not cubicled and we had to trundle heavy, cumbersome

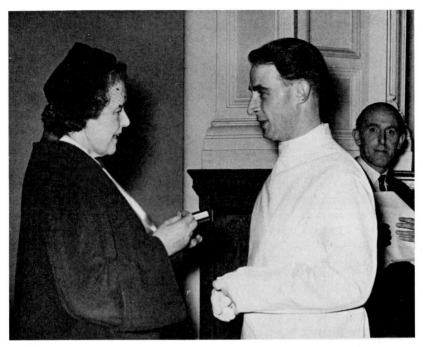

Fig. 62   Bangour Village Hospital Nurses' Prize-giving in 1955. John Sneddon, the first male Gold Medalist receives his medal from the Countess of Rosebery whose ancestor Lord Rosebery officially opened the Hospital in 1906.

screens around to give the patients any privacy. There was a large gym area where a general keep fit class took place most mornings with all the patients exercising all their moveable parts from toes to eyebrows. There was a sunlight room with a central carbon arc lamp (rarely used anywhere in the world nowadays) with goggled patients standing and sitting around in a circle for their treatment session. There were two shortwave machines in a separate room which was surrounded with a mesh screening. A vague explanation for this screening was something to do with interference from or to aeroplanes on their overhead flight paths. Then there was the room containing the large circular bubble bath. The bath was not very deep and the patients sat round the edge enjoying this session. Needless to say, on many occasions the bath was filled with a packet of soap powder producing a huge bubble of frothy suds. There was also the room containing the small bubble bath for use on the arms or legs of individual patients.

The staff room was large and we were joined at coffee time by the ambulance drivers. Most of the patients used the ambulance service because of the distances involved travelling from some of the further corners of West Lothian and there were very few cars on the roads in those days. This was very different from my training days in Liverpool where only patients who were totally immobile or on crutches were transported by ambulance.

In the mornings most of the staff worked in the department, though some spent the full day on the wards at the 'Annexe', as the general hospital was still known at that time. In the afternoon the internal ambulance brought patients from the neurosurgical wards i.e. T1 and T2 in the Annexe and Ward 32 in the Village Hospital to the department for treatment by four of the staff who, later in the afternoon, went with the patients on their return to the ward to treat the patients who were unfit to come to the department. If you were not lucky enough to have the ambulance transport available, you had to walk or take the bus up to the general hospital from the department. Professor Norman Dott was the neurosurgical consultant and operations were carried out in the theatre which was an extension to Ward 32 where there was also a small physiotherapy treatment room. Unfortunately this room was affected by rot and woodworm and had to be demolished.

There have been many changes at the general hospital over the years. 'Q' block was mainly general surgery wards containing a large number of orthopaedic surgical patients. Wards Q7 and Q8 were the eye department and if you worked there as a physiotherapist you were always warned to make sure that the patients didn't cough too much or 'their eyes might end up on their cheeks'! 'P' block was the medical unit with P2 being the pneumonoconiosis ward where the physiotherapists were only able to carry out their treatment on patients if they were able to drag them away from the snooker table which had been installed in the recreation room at the end of the ward. 'R' block was used as a tuberculosis unit mainly filled with pulmonary tuberculosis patients many of whom were nursed outside on the verandahs. This was a very cold job for the physiotherapists when the snow was lying on the ground. One ward in the block was reserved for orthopaedic tuberculosis patients where they rested in their plaster jackets in bed and maintenance physiotherapy was carried out.

Two major operations were carried out each Tuesday and Friday and these patients needed intensive treatment sessions several times a day. Mirrors were fixed to the foot of the patients' bed to help them correct their posture. 'S' block held the maternity unit but there was also a large occupational therapy department where the physiotherapist would sometimes join in the archery sessions held there for the neurosurgical patients in their wheelchairs.

One member of the staff went to Bo'ness and Linlithgow for two or three afternoon and evening sessions of physiotherapy treatment each week. Fortunately a taxi was provided for this journey, in contrast to the journey staff had to make from the Village Hospital to the General Hospital.

The out-patient physiotherapy department moved to wards S3 and 4 in March or April 1956. At that time it was not possible to transfer the bubble baths from Bangour Village Hospital and gradually this form of hydrotherapy treatment fell into disuse. Hydrotherapy was later instituted at the swimming baths in Bathgate and for many years patients were transported by ambulance for their treatment. Eventually the deparment had its own hydrotherapy pool built in 1976.

Miss Nan Watson was appointed Superintendent of the physiotherapy department in 1960 and she held this post until August 1985, at the time of her retirement. Miss Watson was very much responsible for developing an integrated physiotherapy service in Bangour General and Village Hospitals and taking physiotherapy out to the small peripheral hospitals and the community. She was noted as a great organiser and fund raiser and much of the equipment in the physiotherapy department in Bangour General Hospital that is still in use in 1990 was bought as a result of monies raised by Miss Watson.

She recalls with affection how she had been grumbling for many years about the inefficiency of patients and staff having to go by ambulance from Bangour General Hospital physiotherapy department to the swimming pool in Bathgate for hydrotherapy treatment. On one occasion she was making this point at a coffee morning in the company of the late Dr W Reid of Linlithgow who agreed to assist Miss Watson in a fund raising campaign. Dr Reid, The Women's Royal Voluntary Service and Colonel Kidd, who was then Chairman of the Hospital Board of Management, coordinated a magnificent fund raising campaign with Miss Watson and the James T Kidd Memorial Hydrotherapy Pool was opened as an extension to the gym on Ward S4 in 1977. The plaque commemorating the opening of the pool makes special mention of the financial assistance received from the Rotary Club of Linlithgow and Bo'ness, The Linlithgow Ambulance Association and the Women's Royal Voluntary Service (West Lothian District).

Much of Miss Watson's life seems to have been taken up in attending coffee mornings. On another occasion in 1970 she describes meeting Miss Colin Murray who was then Principal of the School of Physiotherapy which has since moved to the Queen Margaret College. On this occasion Miss Watson was successful in persuading the Principal that physiotherapy students should attend Bangour General Hospital physiotherapy department because of the wide range of clinical material that was available for teaching purposes. Subsequently this close link between the School of Physiotherapy and Bangour General Hospital was expanded and in 1978 the Chartered Society of Physiotherapists were happy to recognise the hospital's physiotherapy department as a suitable place to conduct the clinical part of the final examinations that the students had to pass before graduation.

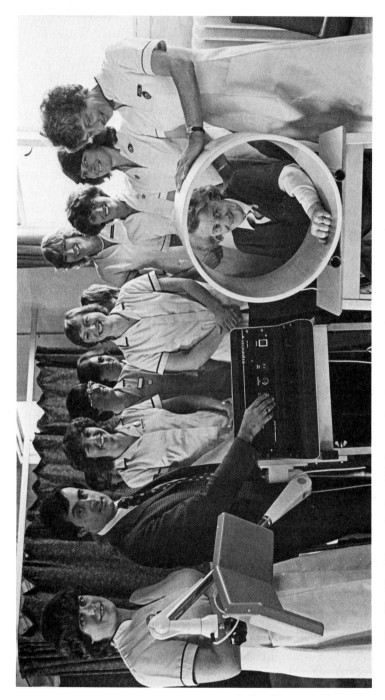

Fig. 63 The Women's Royal Voluntary Services (WRVS) is one of many organisations, businesses and individuals who have presented money or equipment to various departments in the Hospital. Mrs Bunty Hamilton, who organised the WRVS in Bangour for many years, is seen presenting a new piece of equipment to the Physiotherapy Department. John Jack represented the Hospital Management, while Miss Nan Watson (on the right) and her staff enjoy the occasion.

Miss Watson was also involved in the introduction of many innovative treatments in physiotherapy. From the late 1960s Miss Maria Ebner used to come up to Bangour Hospital on an annual basis to conduct courses in connective tissue massage which were attended by physiotherapists from all over the United Kingdom and occasionally courageous members of the medical staff in Bangour General Hospital including Mr A A Gunn and Mr D A D Macleod. Miss Watson and Miss Ebner gained international reputations for the quality of these courses and were invited to present a course in Montreal in 1978. In addition Miss Watson organised many courses on other developments in physiotherapy treatments including Maitland Mobilisation.

In 1981 Miss Watson was entertaining the new consultant physician Dr John Irving to coffee in her office. Dr Irving persuaded Miss Watson and the staff of the department that the time was ripe to develop a Cardiac Rehabilitation Class. Appropriate fund raising took place and staff were trained in a very short time. 'Dr Irving gave us a week to be ready for the first two patients that he had booked in to the very first of these classes.' The Cardiac Rehabilitation Class has developed and expanded over the years but in 1981 it was a very progressive step to take and was well ahead of many other centres in the United Kingdom. A very important part of the class is the exercise patients take in the hydrotherapy pool.

In addition to her fund raising and business activities at coffee mornings, Miss Watson's other main responsibility was to ensure that the social life of the hospital went with a swing. Shortly after she arrived, Miss Watson was asked what she thought of Bangour General Hospital by Jock Milne, Consultant Surgeon. Miss Watson indicated that she thought that it was rather boring and as a result of this comment the physiotherapy annual sports were initiated in 1962 and subsequently were held every year up to 1989 (a total of 27 years), in the grassy area outside the physiotherapy department. Jock Milne undertook the duty of Master of Ceremonies at these sports until his retiral when the Consultant Surgeon who replaced him on the staff, Donald Macleod, took over this aspect of Mr Milne's commitment to Bangour General Hospital life. The sports day was attended by patients and staff from all disciplines, who were encouraged to bring their husbands, wives and children, and much fun was had by all. The highlight of the sports day was always the magnificent tea served by the physiotherapy department, rather than the quality of any of the sporting performances produced on the field. Miss Watson's other main social activity was ensuring that the physiotherapy department hosted a 'Punch Lunch' on Christmas Eve for all hospital staff. This was also a very happy event, frequently being associated with the showing of slides or a video of various members of staff failing to achieve an obviously simple physical feat at the previous summer's sports day. Occasionally the 'Punch Lunch' ended up with the playing of bagpipes and the dancing of Highland reels.

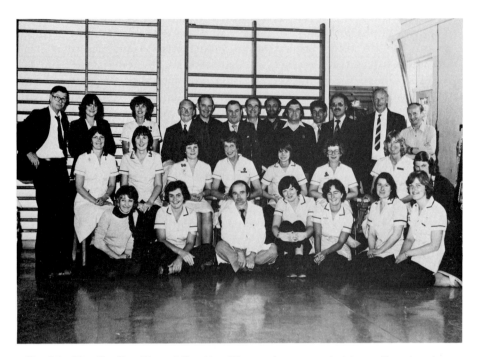

Fig. 64   The Cardiac Class. Miss Nan Watson is surrounded by staff and patients from the Cardiac Rehabilitation Class in the physiotherapy department. Dr John Irving, the Consultant Physician who started the class, is sitting on the floor at Miss Watson's feet.

Miss Watson retired in August 1985 but before she left she had ensured that Jock Milne's physiotherapy clinic for the many orthopaedic patients he treated, had gradually been converted into a Sports Injuries Clinic run by various members of her staff and Mr Donald Macleod. Mr Macleod had developed a great interest in sports injuries as a result of his appointment as Honorary Medical Adviser to the Scottish Rugby Union. Visits of international rugby players to the department for treatment during the international rugby season were, and still are, greatly appreciated by the players and when Scotland won her first Rugby International Grand Slam for sixty years in 1984, a presentation was made by Mr Macleod on behalf of the International Rugby Squad and the Scottish Rugby Union to show their appreciation for the support given to them by the physiotherapy department during that crucial rugby season.

August 1985 saw the arrival of Miss Anne Rankin as Superintendent of the department. Miss Rankin, who had trained in Glasgow and Canada, made many innovative changes to the organisation of the department but has still managed to retain the special happy atmosphere among the staff and to maintain its relationship with other disciplines in the hospital. In addition to reorganising the work load in the department, Miss Rankin has spent a lot of time and effort on the professional development of the physiotherapy staff:

I am firmly of the opinion that a high quality of care requires well educated, well motivated physiotherapists. In addition to developing a staff appraisal programme we now have a continuing in-service training programme and a properly equipped library. In addition I believe that it is important that the department should acquire all the equipment necessary to ensure that patients are being treated to the very highest of modern standards.

In this respect I have taken over Miss Watson's role with regard to fund raising and we have managed to continue to develop the equipment in the department, despite considerable financial restrictions being placed upon us by the Lothian Health Board. The 'Jewel in the Crown' of our fund raising exercise has been the purchase of Kin-Com III, a high tech isokinetic machine which enables us to test and rehabilitate muscles. The Kin-Com was very expensive—£25,000—and I am delighted to report that the community in West Lothian raised £20,000 in fifteen months. The West Lothian Management Team were able to contribute the remaining £5,000. We are justifiably proud that this piece of equipment is available to the patients in West Lothian as the Kin-Com III installed in our department is the very first of its kind in Europe.

Perhaps the greatest development of all has been the introduction of a computerised Physiotherapy Information System and the attempts we have made to measure clinical outcome. This has involved the physiotherapy staff in much extra work and the opportunity to be involved in two major research projects. The first of these projects evaluates the effectiveness of physiotherapy treatment in patients with low back pain by comparing patients treated in a 'back school' with those patients receiving regular treatment on an individual basis. The second project is measuring the effectiveness of physiotherapy treatment for patients who have suffered a stroke. These research projects were developed as a result of the Information System we had established, identifying that 21 per cent of all available physiotherapy time in one year is spent treating stroke patients and 40 per cent of all available time in the out patient department is spent on the treatment of low back pain.

Miss Rankin continues:

We are on the brink of developing a fully comprehensive Information System which will be computer based and will measure both the physiotherapy input to patient care and the results of treatments. This is a very exciting project and yet again I believe that Bangour General Hospital leads the way in research of this type for the whole of the United Kingdom.

In September 1989 Miss Rankin was appointed Unit physiotherapist responsible for integrating the physiotherapy services throughout West Lothian in the hospitals, health centres and schools. Miss Rankin believes that this will ensure a comprehensive and flexible physiotherapy service available to the whole of West Lothian. She concludes:

Our department has been in the fortunate position of being well established over the years and having had good support from both the hospital Management Team and our medical colleagues. The atmosphere in the department is stimulating, highly professional and liberally dosed with humour. I feel we shall never work in an environment like this again. Is it the clapped out wooden huts, the cattle in the fields, Charlie the Donkey, the people of West Lothian or something in the air that has resulted in the development of what I believe is a unique and very special department?

OCCUPATIONAL THERAPY

Work as a rehabilitative measure was first introduced to Bangour Hospital during the First World War when curative workshops were established for the rehabilitation of wounded servicemen. Under the direction of a Royal Engineers Captain, the workshops were equipped and each trade was taught by a qualified craftsman. In the aftermath of the war, mentally ill patients returned to the Village Hospital and benefitted from the opportunities provided by constructive activity and, together with other mental illness hospitals, continued the work under the direction of tradesmen.

The first occupational therapist to practise in the United Kingdom was Miss Margaret Barr Fulton who trained in Philadelphia and took up her appointment in 1925 at the Royal Cornhill Hospital (at that time known as Aberdeen Mental Hospital).

The development of occupational therapy in Edinburgh and its surroundings was the inspiration of Colonel John Cunningham of the Astley Ainslie Hospital, who invited a Canadian, Miss Amy de Brisay, to establish an occupational therapy department in this rehabilitation hospital in 1932. Colonel Cunningham was also responsible for the setting up of the first school of occupational therapy within the Astley Ainslie Hospital in 1939 with an intake of five students.

It was Professor Norman Dott, the early pioneer of surgical neurology, who recognised the unique contribution of occupational therapy at the Astley Ainslie Rehabilitation Hospital and who invited Miss de Brisay to return to Scotland to join his team at Bangour, a team which was truly multi-disciplinary. Professor Dott's weekly case conference, known as 'the blitz', made exciting demands on each team member to contribute, a challenge well met by Miss de Brisay. She made a similar impact in the plastic surgery unit where Mr A B Wallace was treating patients with serious war wounds.

The next significant development of occupational therapy in Bangour was when Dr William Murray's East Lothian Hospital was evacuated to Bangour. Many patients were confined to bed-rest for one year or more and occupational therapy responded to this challenge by planning graded activity, educational programmes and encouragement of social interaction.

In 1945 as the war came to an end, Professor Dott is quoted as saying: 'Among the wartime advances on rehabilitation measures which we were able to secure, the greatest was the return of Miss de Brisay to Scotland and her generous and untiring work with our patients for the cause of rehabilitation in general and occupational therapy in particular. What we owe to her noble and courageous personality and her capable organisation cannot be over-estimated.'

Throughout the wartime years occupational therapy was practised only with the physically disabled, but once the psychiatric patients returned again to the Village, occupational therapy was gradually introduced and for many years surgical neurology and mentally ill patients were both based in the Village Hospital within the same department, Professor Dott seeing the two populations as having similar needs.

In the early 1960s surgical neurology patients transferred to Bangour General Hospital (at that time known as 'the Annexe') and the occupational therapy management of each hospital was organised separately. This facilitated specialisation, which was particularly significant in the Village Hospital where occupational therapists responded to the impact of the development of phenothiazine medication and the opportunities for very specific and constructive rehabilitation and resettlement.

In 1970 the two departments once again came together under a single management structure, and finally in 1986 the first unit head occupational therapist was appointed.

The first department of occupational therapy was housed in Ward 29 of the Village, later to become the Adolescent Unit, and for many years this was the main centre with therapists cycling out to outlying wards and later to the Annexe. In turn, patients were expected to walk or to come by bus from the Annexe to the department in the Village. In the 1950s and 1960s premises were acquired within 'S' block and the psychiatric department moved to the former physiotherapy department. In order to provide premises for industrial work, which was an important treatment medium in that era

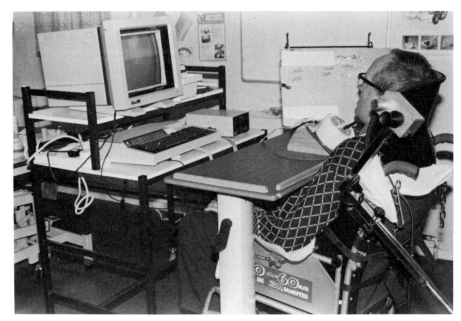

Fig. 65 Computer technology proves a great asset for patients in occupational therapy.

when re-employment in manual work was readily available, a nearby bakery was extensively upgraded. Over the years these buildings were expanded to house a greater variety of activities.

The department of occupational therapy at Bangour Hospital has a significant place in the history of occupational therapy and the part played by Professor Dott in promoting the development of the profession was acknowledged on more than one occasion. He was invited to succeed Colonel Cunningham as President of the former Scottish Association of Occupational Therapy and the Association owes much to his wisdom and guidance at that time. He was later elected an honorary member of that Association. Finally, in 1954 the profession bestowed on Professor Dott its highest honour by appointing him the first advisory fellow of the newly constituted World Federation of Occupational Therapists.

Chapter Thirteen

The Bangour Pioneers

Despite being regarded by some people as being somewhat cut off geo-graphically from the developed world, Bangour has definitely never been cut off from advances in medical practice and it has been the scene of much pioneering work since the beginning of this century, both at the Village Hospital and in the fifty years of life of the General Hospital. These pioneering efforts have included integration of medical care between the community and the hospital, development of occupational therapy, the opening of Scotland's first psychiatric adolescent unit in the community, the role of the computer in clinical practice, innovative work in voice research and management budgeting, to mention just a few fields of activity.

THE LIVINGSTON PROJECT

The unique combination of the beginning of a New Town and the existence of Bangour Village and General Hospitals within five miles of the proposed town centre prompted the Scottish Home and Health Department, in July 1964, to prepare a paper setting out proposals for establishing an integrated health service in Livingston. It is interesting to look at some of the statements in that paper:

> The New Town of Livingston offers a particularly favourable opportunity for planning the co-ordinated development of hospital, local authority and general practitioner services. It has already been agreed that a District Hospital should be established in the New Town, and the object would be to relate the organisation of the other services to this hospital as the central point...it should be possible, with good will all round, to achieve the effect of a combined service in which the demarcation line between hospital and general practice, or between general practice and the local authority services would become of much less significance than it is at present.
> The kind of pattern that might emerge would be a central health services unit consisting of the District Hospital and health centre

accommodation for the local authority and general practitioner services as the focus for all the health services in the New Town, and three or four peripheral health centres providing accommodation for the general practitioner and local authority services and certain hospital facilities. The new pattern would imply appointing doctors with responsibilities both inside and outside hospital and regarding both types of work as the same job.

The Livingston Project was therefore established under the auspices of six authorities working together through a joint advisory committee. The Committee decided that the then vacant post of Medical Superintendent at Bangour General Hospital should be merged with that of Principal Medical Officer to the Livingston Project Advisory Committee. This was more easily said than done for no such post had ever existed before and there were many problems to be resolved before Dr Harry Duncan was able to take up the post with a view to providing creative leadership for the development of the Livingston Health Service Project.

To quote an early report on the project:

The art of maintaining a balance between the community and hospital developments is a vital area in which the Principal Medical Advisor has to play a key role. New job specifications had to be developed for the doctors and others working in the project. Individuals and authorities had to be persuaded to accept new concepts and new ideas and the 'team spirit' had to be fostered, bridging and barriers which existed between the hospital, the local authority health department and the general practitioners.

The report continued

The philosophy of the project which is gradually being implemented, is that so far as is practical and proper, patients should be kept away from hospital and their needs should be met in the community. We have not set out to create a general practitioner/consultant but to steer a middle course between a doctor with a wide but no specialist knowledge and few resources on one hand and a narrow field highly specialised consultant on the other hand. By agreement with the statutory bodies concerned, it was arranged that each general practitioner's list would be limited to about 1,500 patients. For these patients the general practitioner serves as their personal doctor providing the full range of general medical services under the normal Executive Council arrangements. Patients are seen in the health centres by appointment or in their own homes, if necessary. The other half of the conjoint appointment for the general practitioner is a five session commitment with the Regional Hospital Board as a Medical Assistant (later regraded as a Hospital Practitioner) in a speciality. When the general practitioner holding the conjoint appointment is working in the speciality in hospital or community the doctor is then a member of the appropriate consultant team. He is in all senses a member of that consultant speciality team and not in any sense a supernumerary or peripatetic postgraduate student.

One of the crucial influences in developing the project was the need to develop a new role and greater professional satisfaction for general practitioners in the National Health Service. It was thought to be of prime importance in the project that a role be cast for general practitioners that would not only give them personal professional satisfaction to a greater degree but would also redress the balance in terms of prestige between hospital doctors and general practitioners, thus fostering a spirit of professional unity.

Clearly the full development and establishment of this type of practitioner could not be achieved in a brief space of time and it demands not only the production and availability of highly trained young men, but also an attitude of understanding and acceptance amongst the hospital medical staff, so that not only can their skills be utilised to the full but also a real welcome be extended to them by their hospital colleagues. Inevitably the infusion into a district hospital of a number of doctors with conjoint appointments calls for modification of the method of medical staffing within the hospital as well as the community services.

According to the report it was found that the role of the medical assistant varied according to the speciality which was being offered and the initial appointments included general practitioners working in obstetrics and gynaecology, paediatrics, psychiatry, general medicine, ophthalmology and anaesthetics.

The report also stressed that it was equally important to ensure that the Livingston Project was seen to enhance the hospital consultant's role in the community by conducting consultant clinics in health centre premises such as Craigshill, fulfilling the role of postgraduate teacher in his speciality and acting as leader, organiser and pace setter in his speciality in the community.

At first there was only one general practitioner involved in the Livingston Experiment, Dr Hamish Barber, who later went on to become Professor of General Practice in Glasgow University, thanks no doubt in part to his early experiences in West Lothian. By 1968 there were three general practitioners working in the New Town, based in what is now the Craigshill Health Centre and the doctors in post in the early days included Dr D G Bain, Dr W J Bassett and Dr F I Stewart working in paediatrics; Dr I C Buchan, Dr C M Corser and Dr J McMichael working in psychiatry; Dr J W Davie and Dr M Gardner working in general medicine/geriatrics; Dr H D R Munro working in obstetrics and gynaecology; Dr B M Moore in ophthalmology and Dr Margaret Riddoch in anaesthetics. Two other doctors, as well as Dr

Barber, had already left the scheme by 1973 and they were Dr F Hayes who went to work full-time in industrial medicine and Dr A J Haines who accepted a post as Director of Student Health Services for Polytechnic colleges in North London.

Since there were no doctors ready made for this type of general practitioner/hospital speciality conjoint appointment it was necessary to set up a vocational training scheme. The aim of this scheme was to appoint young doctors who would have been graduated for about two years and they would then spend at least one year in general practice, one year in the speciality in which the doctor ultimately hoped to practice, six months in general medicine and a further six months obtaining experience in other specialities according to the doctor's needs and interests. Appointment to the vocational training scheme did not automatically guarantee an appointment in Livingston as a principal in general practice but in any event it was believed that completion of the programme would produce a well trained general practitioner ready to commence practice in any part of the country. During the period 1968–1972 ten doctors took part in this vocational training scheme and it was subsequently expanded in April 1984 to apply to general practitioner training programmes throughout the Lothian Region.

The main driving forces stimulating the development of the Livingston Project in its early days were Sir John Brotherson who was then the Chief Medical Officer in the Scottish Home and Health Department, supported by Mr John Gibb as Chairman of the Health Services Joint Advisory Committee for the Livingston Area, and Dr Andrew Duncan, the Principal Medical Officer on the Advisory Committee who also undertook the post of Medical Superintendent at Bangour General Hospital.

In the Scottish Home and Health Department report of 1973 these individuals were able to note that the principle sources of satisfaction behind the Livingston project were:

- The high quality of doctors recruited.
- The degree to which the conjoint general practitioner/hospital specialist has succeeded in practice despite the built-in theoretical difficulties of (a) conflicting claims on time between community and speciality and (b) acceptance in the specialities by the consultants.
- The vocational training scheme and the high quality of its recruits, the changing and encouraging attitude of hospital consultants to the project and to the conjoint appointment.

Various disappointments and areas of concern were also identified in the report including:

- Failure to integrate adequately, at that time, the hospital and general practice services with the school health service, social work, occupational health, and nursing.

All of these areas of concern have subsequently been addressed.
Dr Ross Munro reported in 1989 that:

In the 25 years that have passed since the start of the Livingston Project the role of the general practitioner in the community has changed greatly, making it more and more difficult to make the scheme work. Time is the great enemy. No matter what happens in general practice a doctor who holds a hospital practitioner appointment simply cannot phone Bangour and say that he is not coming.

On the hospital side, Bangour ran out of the need for more specialist hospital practitioners after the specialities involved had expanded to include the Accident and Emergency Department. The population of Livingston kept on growing, demanding more general practitioners, so several have now had to be appointed as full time in general practice without a hospital speciality. Accordingly we now have many health centres in Livingston where the hospital practitioner scheme has become diluted although, this in itself does not detract from the valuable role that the GP hospital practitioners play in the community.

I still think it gives general practitioners an opportunity to develop a special interest while the hospital benefits by gaining mature doctors who make a regular long term service commitment to a speciality which hospital trainees in Registrar and Senior Registrar appointments can never provide.

I believe that the Livingston Scheme has provided a service to the hospital department in which it has been involved as well as working well in some areas in the community. The primary care teams of general practitioners in the New Town have developed nursing teams which include midwives and this helps integrate care when local mothers come into the maternity unit of Bangour and more recently St John's Hospital. Tremendous advances have also taken place with regard to the care of psychiatric patients in the community and the development of psychological support services based at the health centres.

I believe these outcomes are a great compliment to the original vision contained in the Livingston Health Service Project and all credit must be given to those in the various medical services who have persevered to make the idea at least partially a reality.

One of the most interesting areas in which to study the implementation of the Livingston Health Service Project is in the field of paediatrics. At the time the project was being initiated in 1968, Dr Gordon Stark was appointed consultant paediatrician for West Lothian. Prior to this date the only specialist paediatric services in West Lothian had been twice weekly visits to the newborn nursery by staff from the

Royal Hospital for Sick Children in Edinburgh and a follow-up out patient clinic for babies.

In a paper delivered at a symposium held in Livingston in 1971, Dr W J Bassett wrote:

It is accepted and believed by the Health Centre Team at Craigshill that the future of child health practice depends on the principle of child care being based within the community. There is a need to produce an integrated system of care which will do away with much of the present waste of resources.

Over the years, five general practitioners have held conjoint appointments as either medical assistants or hospital practitioners in the speciality of paediatrics in Bangour General Hospital and St John's Hospital at Howden. To be appointed a hospital practitioner in a speciality the practitioner concerned must be trained to such a standard that he has spent up to two years in the relevant speciality or has appropriate post graduate qualifications which take about the same time to achieve. In addition the practitioner must hold an appointment as a principal in general practice. In 1989 there were four GP hospital practitioners in paediatrics—Dr W Bassett, Dr F Stewart, Dr F Shah and Dr J Handley.

Dr Stark and his team were responsible for continuing the follow-up baby clinic at Bangour General Hospital and developing a general medical paediatric out patient clinic based in the hospital. In due course the consultant paediatric surgeons from the Western General Hospital in Edinburgh were also able to develop a surgical paediatric out patient clinic in Bangour.

A policy of 'outreach paediatrics' was steadily developed. The GP hospital practitioners held paediatric clinics in the Livingston Health Centres on a fortnightly basis, seeing children referred by their GP colleagues or referred from hospital for follow-up. The consultant also ran a clinic in each health centre once a month. These outreach clinics were also developed in areas of West Lothian other than Livingston including Broxburn, Fauldhouse, Whitburn and Bathgate.

The needs of handicapped children received special attention. Dr Stark encouraged Dr F Stewart to develop a special interest as a hospital practitioner in the very difficult area of caring for the handicapped child. Together they ran clinics in the four special schools in West Lothian in conjunction with the school doctor and, when appropriate, the physiotherapist and speech therapist would also take part.

Long before West Lothian had a hospital orthopaedic service there were children's orthopaedic clinics held in various parts of the region, closely associated with the community physiotherapy service which was particularly well-developed. A combined clinic was established, run jointly by the pae-diatricians and Mr W Anderson the orthopaedic surgeon. This valuable service was particularly important for children with cerebral palsy. The pae-diatric department, as a result of good communications between the hospital practitioners, the school health service and community services, was able to establish close working relationships with Barnardo's Family Support Teams, the social work department, the Royal Scottish Society for the Prevention of Cruelty to Children and the many other agencies in West Lothian involved in meeting the needs of children.

During the 1970s and 1980s considerable advances were taking place in the care of new born babies and in particular premature babies. With approximately 2,000 deliveries per year the obstetric unit at Bangour was the second busiest in Lothian. Paediatric services were gradually expanded to cope with the care of these babies. Whereas previously the medical care of the newborn had largely been in the hands of resident doctors in the obstetric department, senior house officers were now appointed full time within the hospital paediatric department to cope with the increasing demands and complexity of the work. The staffing of a neonatal unit without an associated general paediatric in-patient ward presented considerable difficulties both in providing an adequate range of experience for hospital doctors and nurses in training, and in providing middle and senior grade medical cover. Dr Frank Stewart and Dr F Shah both played a very important role in the work of the neonatal unit and it is impossible to estimate the overall contribution made to this particular aspect of paediatric care in West Lothian by the four hospital practitioners.

Valuable support was received for the neonatal unit by the regional intensive neonatal care unit at the Simpson Memorial Maternity Hospital in Edinburgh. Particularly ill or premature babies were transferred there if necessary, either in a transport incubator or, preferably, in the best incubator of all, in the mother's womb before birth, if a set of hazardous circumstances had been identified in advance.

The community in West Lothian has always been particularly proud of its neonatal unit and has participated in many fund raising exercises designed to ensure that any baby born in West Lothian has the benefit of the very best facilities available.

The inclusion of West Lothian in the rotational training scheme for medical paediatric registrars provided an unusual opportunity for middle grade hospital staff to gain experience of work in the school medical service and other community child services, in addition to providing additional support for the neonatal unit.

The whole concept of the original Livingston Project was to ensure that the children of West Lothian received a high standard of integrated care, linking the services provided by the community, general practice and the hospital. This ambition received a tremendous boost when, as a result of a question raised in the House of Commons by Mr Robin Cook, MP for Livingston, the then Under Secretary of State for Scotland responsible for Health Services announced that there would be a paediatric ward in the new Livingston Hospital. This important development had been eagerly discussed for many years and was the subject of tremendous public interest among the community in West Lothian. The announcement was received with enthusiasm throughout West Lothian.

Over the last twenty-five years of the Livingston Project, the challenges facing paediatrics and the development of integrated child health care in West Lothian have changed. The social and educational needs of children have assumed increasing importance together with the provision of first class medical care through the integrated paediatric services. A significant contribution has been made by general practitioners holding conjoint hospital practitioner appointments in paediatrics.

COMPUTERS ARE HERE TO STAY

Why use computers in hospital? At the same time as life expectancy of the general population has increased, there has been a planned and rapid increase in the number of people living and working in West Lothian. Patients coming to hospital have increasingly sophisticated expectations of how they will be received and their problem resolved following a series of investigations and treatment which may involve several different specialities and departments. This co-ordination of effort places great demands on the medical staff to ensure that administrative pathways function smoothly to allow them to do their work. It has been estimated that a surgeon requires a support team of up to thirty-five other individuals before he can undertake even the most straightforward minor operation on a patient.

It has become apparent that the co-ordination of clinical work and administrative services requires a highly sophisticated computerised support system. Indeed computers have become vital tools in the day to day work of many of the departments at the Bangour Hospitals.

Mrs Elizabeth Lumsden recalls:

When I first took up my post as Adviser in Computer Services in 1983 there were, at that time eight computers based in six different departments in Bangour General Hospital. In the subsequent six years the number of computers and sites on which they can be found has grown so dramatically that they seem to be flourishing like the cones on a motorway.

I will try to highlight some of the different stages of the growth and spread of their use through the hospital as that gives an idea of how dependent we have all become on computer technology. In addition I will try to point out those fields in which Bangour General Hospital has been the pioneer, mainly due to the dedication and imaginative thinking of the staff in the relevant departments.

One of the earliest 'firsts' was the installation, in 1976 by Mr Tony Gunn, the Consultant Surgeon, of a micro computer system (which has had to be updated twice), in the Accident and Emergency Department. This computer was used to record the symptoms and signs of abdominal pain in those patients who came up to the department on a standard document which would then have the information fed into the computer by the receiving junior doctor. The computer, programmed to collate information on the signs and symptoms of previous patients, then produces data giving an indication in percentage terms of what disease the patient could be suffering from. For example, the computer might suggest that there was a 99 per cent probability of the patient having acute appendicitis or alternatively a 75 per cent probability of having non-specific abdominal pain. The discipline of having to fill in a structured case note, which is then fed into the computer and subsequently reviewed by the senior medical staff, rapidly increases the accuracy and confidence of junior doctors in assessing patients with abdominal pain and as a result fewer are admitted to hospital and fewer have unnecessary operations. Accordingly the installation of the computer has been instrumental in saving the National Health Service hundreds of thousands of pounds and in addition has saved a lot of patients from needless suffering and unnecessary operations.

December 1981 saw the introduction of the first 'scientific' computer which was, and still is, being used to record the results from the machines used in the Biochemistry laboratory for analysis of blood and urine. As a result of the computerised system the patients' samples are handled much more quickly and the results are printed rather than hand written, so there is no danger that the doctors writing can be misinterpreted when the results reach the ward or the patient's own general practitioner.

The general surgical department in Bangour Hospital has participated in the Edinburgh Surgical Audit for many many years. In the early 1980s, because of Mr Tony Gunn's expertise with computers and his interest in audit, Bangour became one if the first units participating in the Edinburgh Surgical Audit to be computerised. Information is recorded about the number and type of operations carried out in the surgical unit and the results are collected once a year for audit and for comparison with similar surgical departments in other hospitals. As the result of these audit studies, a significant increase in specialisation of patient care has taken place, the best known example being the development of the speciality of vascular surgery and surgical urology. In this way the standards of patient care are increased by concentrating

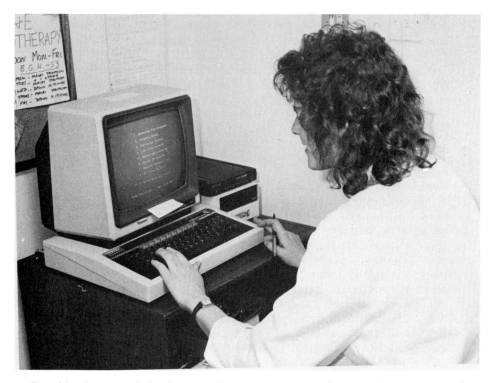

Fig. 66 A young lady doctor using a computer to improve the accuracy of
diagnosing abdominal pains such as appendicitis.

patients with similar problems in departments with appropriate surgical
skills to deal with them.

Another 'first for Britain' for Bangour, although admittedly only by
a few days, was the installation and subsequent use in 1983 of a
Viewdata Terminal in the Accident and Emergency Department allowing doctors and nurses to link directly to the world famous Poisons
Bureau in Edinburgh. The staff in the Accident and Emergency
Department had immediate access to the best possible advice about
the correct antidote and treatment when a patient was admitted as a
result of a drug overdose or accidental poisoning with a household or
gardening chemical such as paraquat. In this way precious minutes
could be saved, thus increasing the chance of the patients survival.

One of the first administrative computer systems to be installed
occurred in 1982 when Mr David Bolton and his staff in the Pharmacy
department installed their own computer to run a stock management
programme in the Pharmacy stores department. The hospital engineers,
who are based down in Bangour Village Hospital, pioneered the use
of a Works Management Information System, whereby the computer

is used to record the progress and costing of work throughout the hospital complex as well as providing other information necessary for effective management.

From 1984 computers started to mushroom, one of the next major systems being installed in the x-ray department. As the result of the hard work and dedication of Dr Ian Parker, the software to run a patient record system was devised which, since its introduction, speeds up the progress of the reporting of x-rays so that patients and doctors get the results much more quickly. The system also keeps figures for the annual statistical return which are then used to ensure that the most efficient use is being made of staff. Following one particular study the hours of duty of the radiographers were adjusted to meet demand placed on the department by patients coming from general practitioners to have x-rays taken. Providing this type of service to general practice is greatly appreciated by patients and doctors throughout West Lothian but it is important that the pressures this places on the department are minimised by ensuring an even spread of workload throughout the day from 8.30 a.m. till 7.00 p.m.

The year 1985 was memorable in the computing history of Bangour for two reasons. This was the year when Bangour was invited, along with Inverclyde Royal in Greenock, to become a pilot site for the introduction of Management Budgeting to Scotland. The exact cost of every aspect of patient care was to be analysed in the hope that it would be possible to identify areas where money could be better spent. Unfortunately this pilot scheme was unsuccessful and abandoned after two or three years. The cost of introducing this scheme and the commitment required by all the staff involved in the pilot study had been underestimated. There were areas of success such as the x-ray department, Pharmacy, physiotherapy department and to a lesser extent nursing and laboratory medicine. There were no real successes with this pilot scheme as far as the medical staff were concerned, in that accurate costs of the different treatments offered to patients were never identified.

The second big event in 1985 was the installation of an integrated hospital information system known as HOMER. Much research was carried out to try to find the most appropriate system for the hospital, including sending a team of investigators all the way to Australia, under the leadership of the then District Administrator Mr Alec Maltman. The whole concept behind HOMER is that basic details of the patient—name, age, sex, home address, occupation, general practitioner etc—need only be recorded once, and at any subsequent hospital visit or admission this information is already available to the staff from the computer memory, thus saving a lot of time wasting and repetitive recordings of details.

We've looked at the role of computers in patient care and administration. Many people still think of computers as being used for playing games and indeed this also takes place in the hospital in that

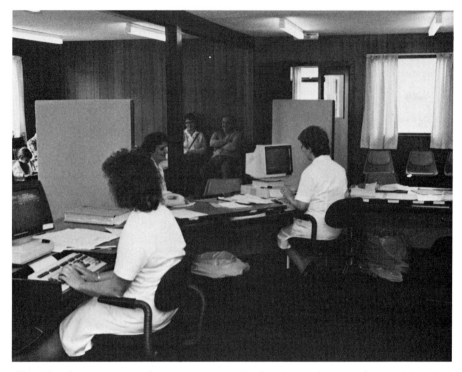

Fig. 67 Computers are here to stay—and take the strain out of organising the admission of patients to hospital once their personal details are entered into the Patient Information System.

the patients in the occupational therapy department and paediatric clinics can participate in a variety of educational and entertaining games to help them enjoy their time in hospital.

Computerisation is here to stay. Hospital staff, irrespective of their speciality or department will, in the future, spend increasing time with personal desk top computers, hopefully taking up less time than used to be devoted to making hand written notes on paper.

THE ADOLESCENT UNIT

Bangour's Adolescent Unit, which opened in October 1957, was very much a pioneering effort being the first in Scotland. For some time Dr (later Professor) A K M Macrae, the Hospital Superintendent, and Dr B E A Magill, Consultant Psychiatrist, had been convinced that it was necessary to remove from the adult wards the ever increasing number of adolescent patients being treated at the Village Hospital. They therefore travelled to England hoping to learn from existing units which worked with teenagers. They returned unimpressed, however, as all the units they visited were locked, with custody given priority over therapy for the disturbed young patients. Secure accommodation, solitary confinement and even cells were completely contrary to the Bangour tradition of treatment and so, with the complete support of Dr Macrae, Dr Betty Magill, as Consultant responsible for the new venture, decided that the Adolescent Unit should be entirely open and without locked doors, far less bars. The Unit took over the former fever isolation Ward 31 where, with only minimal alterations and additions it has operated successfully for over thirty years. The accommodation was shaped like a butterfly with the two wings each housing small wards of eight beds, one for boys, the other for girls. The central sunny rooms provided for both a lounge and dining-room which allowed the sexes to mix together throughout the day. There was no room in the building for a school and this was therefore placed in a separate building within the Village Hospital grounds some half a mile away from the Unit. This was seen as a positive advantage as it meant that the adolescents had to go out to school just like any other teenagers and the walk allowed time to defuse any rows or upsets which may have occurred early in the morning.

So novel was the whole concept that young patients soon began to arrive from all over Scotland and the North of England. Most of the youngsters, whose ages ranged from 12 years to 16 years, were suffering from emotional and neurotic disorders but some presented as a result of psychotic or organic problems.

From the outset an approach was adopted which encouraged the young patients to talk to each other and try to understand one another's problems. This therapeutic community approach was to prove most successful. The nursing staff at the Bangour Adolescent Unit were actively encouraged to take their young patients out and trips to the swimming pool in Bathgate and visits to local shops were often organised. This open approach, unheard of in existing English units, often led to teenagers being able to return home sooner, and the average length of stay in the unit was reduced to under six months. Eventually, all members of staff in the Adolescent Unit happily wore civvies rather than uniforms and encouraged the teenagers to address them on first name terms.

The informality successfully adopted at Bangour has been intentionally developed over the years. In 1976 Dr Pamela Wills was appointed as the first fully trained Child and Adolescent Psychiatrist to the Unit, and in 1979 Dr John Aspin became the Consultant in charge having been trained in the Young People's Unit in Edinburgh. Changes to the philosophy of the Unit have been assisted by the continuity of service of many of the staff involved, such as Nursing Assistant Jean Hughes who joined the Unit staff when it first opened, and Ward Sister Anne Macrae who has worked there for over twenty years. Whilst others worried that the informality of the atmosphere might lead to a loss of authority, the staff, under Dr Aspin's guidance, have confidently used this approach without any resulting loss of control. The success of the Unit was such that over the past decade it became apparent that the natural progression would be away from the hospital setting altogether and into the community itself. Such a move would remove the stigma of admission to a mental hospital for young people, a factor which could have a considerable bearing on the development of youngsters at a crucial time in their lives. Providing care in the community would also mean that young people would be much less cut off from family and friends. Much of the pioneering work in group therapy both in the Unit and the community was started at Bangour by Charge Nurse Duncan Tennant who has been appointed as the hospital's only Nurse Therapist to date. Many of his efforts have been directed at secondary school age youngsters with the aim of providing preventive group therapy within schools thus, it is hoped, removing the need for residential treatment at a later date.

Given its community orientation, it was very appropriate that the Adolescent Unit should, in the summer of 1989, be the first department to move to Livingston from Bangour; not to St John's at Howden however, but to its own site at Willowgrove, Craigshill. The acceptance of the Unit by the community was not gained without some difficulty. It says much for the way in which Dr Aspin and his dedicated staff have gone about involving the Livingston Development Corporation officials and members of the public that the confidence and co-operation of the Unit's new neighbours in Willowgrove was gained. So integrated into the local community has the Unit become that from the outside it looks just like any other block of flats. Inside, the accommodation has been skilfully converted to meet the residential and educational needs of the children in an attractive way while still incorporating most up to date technology.

RADIOLOGY

Miss Margaret Barr started work as a radiographer in Bangour Hospital in 1947 when the staff consisted of three radiographers and one student. There was a visiting Radiologist, Dr Robert Saffley, who reported on the films and carried out some special examinations such as barium meals. In 1948 10,000 patients were examined.

Miss Barr recalls that

> the early years were memorable for our work for Professor Norman Dott, Neurosurgeon, who operated in the theatre in Ward 32 in Bangour Village Hospital. X-rays were taken during the course of

many of these operations using a very basic low powered mobile machine. Somehow we managed to produce good stereoscopic views of the brain, taking at least sixteen films of 2–3 seconds exposure each. This required a degree of versatility and improvisation unknown in the present days of high technology.

There was also a general x-ray room situated in Village Wards 3 and 4 which was used one evening a week when Mr Noel Gray and Mr Jock Milne held their surgical out patient clinics there. This would be the original x-ray department before the Annexe or General Hospital was built.

Miss Barr continues:

the main x-ray department was in 'R' block and had a good all round diagnostic unit donated by the American Red Cross and a small mobile unit for use in the wards. This machine was truly 'portable'. It had also been donated by the Americans and the descriptive literature that came with it confirmed that the machine was capable of being 'dropped by parachute without detriment'. In my time in West Lothian we never put it to the test.

In the 1940s and early 1950s the work in the General Hospital was largely with patients suffering from spinal and pulmonary tuberculosis. It was heavy work dealing with these patients as they came to the x-ray department in a complete plaster cast and had to be lifted out and moved onto the x-ray tables with great care. Some of the chest patients reported for x-ray each week, to have their treatment assessed and at follow up clinics there would be a queue of up to seventy patients waiting for attention. We got to know many of these patients very well and had a real interest in following their progress.

At this time, improvisation was the antecedent of modern technology and engineering invention: patients undergoing certain examination of the lungs had to be angled 45° head down on the x-ray table. I have a vivid memory of all the staff available hanging on to an arm or a leg or some other part of the patient's anatomy to keep him from sliding head first off the table while the consultant physician counted out the delay before the films were to be taken in lugubrious tones— '1 dead donkey, 2 dead donkeys, 3 dead donkeys'—right up to the necessary '20 dead donkeys' or 20 seconds when the staff and patient were able to draw breath again once the x-ray had been taken.

In these days there was no official 'on call' system and certainly no extra payment. It was part of the job and generally the only calls for x-rays out of normal working hours were from Professor Dott's unit. The radiographer in the Village had to live in the nurses' home to be ready for a quick sprint to Ward 32.

My first ever call out to the General Hospital was for a child with a suspected broken leg. I was visiting friends in the Newington district of Edinburgh. Very few staff had cars in those early days and I had to take a tram to St Andrew's Square and a bus to the main gate of the Village Hospital. It was pitch dark by this time so I went to the Village Nurses' Home to collect a torch and then walked up to the General Hospital.

Soon after that in 1969 the new Casualty Department was opened in Ward Q1 and the new x-ray department in Q2. The staff had increased to seven radiographers with a supporting secretarial and dark room staff and a full on call/stand by service was initiated. This was necessary because of the terrible increase in traffic accidents that had taken place on the Edinburgh/Glasgow road which was known as the Horror Highway with its unenviable reputation of having the highest accident rate of any road in the British Isles. In radiography circles our department was regarded as highly experienced in dealing with victims of these accidents, many of which produced very bizarre injuries to the head, face and neck and this was before the days of seat belts. I well remember attending a lecture in another hospital on head injuries by an eminent South of England surgeon and feeling considerable annoyance as he proudly showed, with no acknowledgement of its source, a picture of a very unusual head injury, an x-ray film taken by myself at Bangour Hospital several years earlier!

In 1968 the total number of patients examined in the x-ray department had risen to 26,000 from 10,000 in 1948. Dr Kenneth Wood was appointed Consultant Radiologist at that time to assist Dr Robert Saffley in coping with this major work load. Dr Saffley retired in 1974 to be replaced initially by Dr Alastair McKintosh in 1979. Dr McKintosh subsequently left and the consultant staff in the department was increased to three with the appointments of Dr Ian Parker and Dr Peter Reddy to support Dr Wood in dealing with the ever increasing number of patients requiring x-ray examination.

Miss Barr believes that it was the introduction of the automatic film processor which revolutionised the work of the x-ray department in the early 1970s. Gone were the days of the dark room with its open tanks and evil smelling chemicals, producing wet films after a wait of 15 minutes or so. Many a young radiographer and member of the junior medical staff had spent a happy few minutes in the dark room waiting for these films! The development of automatic film processors saw the end of the poor patients having to walk or be wheeled up and down the corridors of the hospital clutching wet x-ray films which would eventually be returned to the department all stuck together in the hope that they could then be accurately reported by the Radiologist. Nowadays it is possible to produce an x-ray picture completely processed, dried and ready for reporting in 90 seconds.

An important expansion of the x-ray service was the opening of the ultra sound department at the end of the 1970s, providing a service which was well used particularly by the maternity unit, but also for many other medical

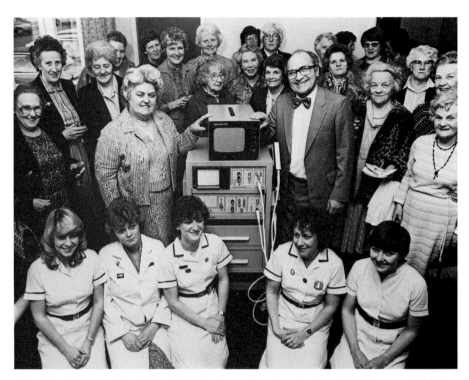

Fig. 68 The people of West Lothian have been unstinting in their support of the Bangour Hospitals. The Women's Rural Institute present an ultrasound 'baby scanner' to the X-ray Department. Sandy Findlay, Chairman of the Lothian Health Board accepts the gift on behalf of a group of radiographers. At the same time, the WRI raised money for a Mammogram machine used in the early detection of breast cancer.

examinations. The West Lothian Women's Rural Institute organised a massive fund raising appeal in 1982, raising over £21,000 for a mammography unit and an additional ultra sound scanner.

In the 1980s the x-ray department, with its staff of three Consultant Radiologists, fourteen radiographers and appropriate supporting secretarial and technical staff, was a well-equipped up-to-date unit able to supply the services required by modern medical practice. In addition, the department, under the guidance of Dr Ian Parker, embarked on a programme of computerisation of the patients' records, examinations carried out and the underlying costs of running the department. At the present time the number of patients attending the department has reached a total of 50,000 every year compared to the 10,000 patients examined in 1948. These 50,000 people amount to 1 in 3 of the population of West Lothian.

Miss Barr concluded her comments about the expansion of x-ray services in West Lothian by commenting at the time of her retiral in 1989, shortly before the department moved to St John's Hospital, that during her working life the department had developed beyond all recognition and 'there are no more dead donkeys'.

PHARMACY

Another department that has grown beyond recognition is Pharmacy. First mention of the Dispensary or Pharmacy at Bangour is documented at the time of the conversion of Bangour Village Hospital to the Edinburgh War Hospital in 1914, when it is recorded that 'the resources of the dispensary of the mental hospital were supplemented by stores for reserves of drugs, dressings, instruments and appliances and a splint store'.

After psychiatric patients returned to the Village Hospital in 1923, their medicinal needs were met by the services of one dispenser, as Miss Margaret Allister was then described. By 1927 the title of Pharmacist was in use and the post at that time was filled by Miss Christian B M Cleghorn.

After the opening of the hutted annexe during the Second World War, Pharmacy still remained a one-man show. The first Pharmacist to occupy the single room dispensary in 'P' block was a Mr Lumsden who later left this specialty to train as a general practitioner. He was succeeded by Miss Sheila Gardner who continued to provide a complete Pharmacy service single-handed until 1945.

> We had very few drugs available [recalls Miss Gardner], but what stores we had were kept under lock and key and I'll never forget the huge bunch of keys which I had to carry around. I was provided with the services of one of the male patients from the Village Hospital, who had been kept at Bangour during the war to work as a porter while the other men and the staff were away fighting. At first I was very apprehensive about going down into the cellar to fetch supplies with him, but I always found him most co-operative and helpful.

Even out of evil, good can sometimes come and one benefit which resulted from the research carried out during the Second World War was the increasing availability of powerful drugs, including the development of Penicillin, but even by 1948 the total expenditure for pharmaceutical services was only £27,000. The discovery and use of Streptomycin in the fight against tuberculosis was a major breakthrough and helped to account for the increase in Bangour's pharmacy budget to £45,000 in 1957. To put these figures into proportion it is interesting to note that the total bill, in 1989, for providing drugs, dressings and incontinence products for the Bangour Village and General Hospitals was approximately £1.26 million.

In the mid 1950s a sterile syringe service was operational throughout the United Kingdom, supplied by Hospital Instruments, a subsidiary of Smith and Nephew, a company well known for the manufacture of elastoplast. The syringes at that time were glass and came in individual containers sealed with wax and these containers were capped. Estimates of usage were made and Hospital Instruments brought an initial delivery of an agreed quantity of syringes in various sizes; once a week the company was informed of the number of syringes used and they then provided a topping up service on a one-for-one basis. This service stopped around 1959 by which time the Pharmacy began supplying disposable syringes and needles. In the late 1950s when a Mrs Carus was the Principal Pharmacist a start was made on a central sterile service in the hospital. The Occupational Therapy Industrial Unit came into being at that time, the first in Scotland, and Bangour General Hospital had the first sterile procedure pack service within any hospital in Scotland. After liaising with the doctors and nurses as to what was required, raw materials were supplied to the Occupational Therapy Department who made them up into packs for use on the wards and operating theatres. That type of sterile supply service carried on for four or five years until proprietary commercial packs were introduced about 1964–5.

Mr John Russell was appointed Chief Pharmacist in Bangour in 1962 and he comments that the development of commercial disposable syringes and needles, procedure packs and sterile supply services was associated with a dramatic increase in expenditure in the Bangour Pharmacy Department. It also led to a considerable reduction in the diversity of packs which were made up in the Occupational Therapy Industrial Unit, limiting them to those packs which were originally designed for the Burns Unit such as the sterile gamgee and bandages pack.

These various developments were mainly supervised by Mr Jim Strachan who was appointed to the Pharmacy Department in 1956 in the specific role of organising Pharmacy purchasing at the General Hospital. He retired in 1988 having spent thirty-two years developing the Pharmacy Supplies and Stores so that they ran like clockwork and no ward sister was ever stuck for an essential piece of equipment. It was not all work for Mr Strachan in the Pharmacy Stores in that he managed to meet and marry his wife when she was a student training in Bangour Hospital.

It was during Mr J Russell's time as Principal Pharmacist that sterile production of drugs was introduced to the Pharmacy Department such as making eyedrops and special intravenous infusions. Mr David Bolton took over from Mr Russell in 1978 and at that time a portacabin was built on to the Pharmacy Department and this area was developed into a sophisticated sterile production service. This portacabin or prefabricated unit was one of the first such units designed for any Pharmacy Department to be produced in the United Kingdom. Subsequent to it being opened, visitors from all over the United Kingdom and the Middle East visited the unit and its design has been adopted in many different parts of the world. In addition, soon after it was commissioned, the unit was used to produce the first large volume 3 litre intravenous total parenteral nutrition solutions used within the Lothian Health Board. Early in 1983 the unit produced the first 3 litre total parenteral nutrition solutions containing fat emulsion for administration as a single unit to debilitated patients. To our knowledge this is the first time such a solution has ever been prepared in Scotland.

Returning to the 1950s, on the Psychiatric side in Bangour Village Hospital there were very few preparations in general use; most of the medication supplied to the Village Hospital took the form of paraldehyde drafts which proved to be a very effective sedative but had an awful smell. Every day the Pharmacy issued 150 to 200 doses of the draft in 2 oz bottles containing about 5 mls of paraldehyde and 2 ozs of water. This was very inexpensive and it was not until about 1955 or 1956 that more expensive medications for treating psychiatric patients came into general use—chlorpromazine (largactil), thioridazine (melleril) etc. This led to a tremendous increase in Pharmacy expenditure.

Also in the early 1950s, the main group of patients in the General Hospital had tuberculosis and they were housed in 'R' block. There were upwards of 200 tuberculosis patients in the hospital at that time. They were long-stay patients and again the drug treatment they received was comparatively inexpensive being para-aminosalicylic acid (PAS) and one or two other preparations such as streptomycin or isoniazid. In the General Hospital at that time, apart from penicillin injections being used on virtually every patient who had surgery, a sort of umbrella treatment which often created more problems than it solved, there was not a wide range of pharmaceutical products used. The same cannot be said about the vast range of medications that have been developed and are now used throughout the hospital. Following discussions between Mr J Russell and Mr David Bolton, who took over as Principal Pharmacist, and senior medical staff in Bangour Village and General Hospital, the West Lothian Drug and Therapeutics Committee was established in around 1976. This committee has representatives from the Pharmacy Department as well as the Village and General Hospitals and nursing. In addition the General Practitioners were represented on the committee as well as the hospital administration and treasurer. This committee felt that its main responsibility was to objectively assess any new drug as it came on the market with a view to ensuring that the patients in West Lothian got the very best treatment, while keeping Pharmacy costs under control. The committee, which was initially chaired by Dr A Wright, and then by Mr Donald Macleod from 1978 to 1990, proved very effective in that it developed the first working hospital drug formulary in any of the Lothian Health Board Hospitals. This formulary acted as an educational tool to all the doctors in West Lothian, both junior and senior, by giving guidance as to what had been agreed to be the most effective first line treatment for a vast majority of commonly encountered medical and surgical problems. The formulary proved to be of particular value in the control of the introduction of very skilfully marketed products, such as antibiotics of which there seemed to be more and more developed every day of the week. In addition, Bob McCartney, during his time as Drug Information Services Pharmacist in Bangour Hospital, designed a first class '*HITCH-HIKERS GUIDE TO DRUG ADVERTISING*' to help doctors read and understand the promotional literature produced by drug companies so that they could sift out those drugs which would be of genuine value to their patients.

These efforts, supplemented by a daily visit from the Pharmacist to the wards throughout the hospital, helped ensure that Bangour Pharmacy lived within its drug budget for most of the 1980s—a remarkable achievement.

The Pharmacy Department in Bangour was involved in computerisation of its drug services from 1976 onwards and it was one of Mr David Bolton's proud boasts, before he left West Lothian to become Chief Administrative Pharmaceutical Officer or the Lothian Health Board, that he could trace every individual paracetamol tablet from the moment it arrived in his department until it was swallowed by an individual patient in the ward—another unique achievement in a forward looking department which is being led into the 1990s by its new Principal Pharmacist, Mr Grant Nicol.

THE BANGOUR LABORATORIES

Hospital laboratories carry out tests on body fluids and tissues which form the modern scientific basis for making a diagnosis and assessing the patient's progress. Its staff represent 'the back-room boys' of the hospital service, providing vital diagnostic information to the doctors yet they are rarely seen by the patient, who may well be unaware of their existence. This subject includes several different but sometimes overlapping disciplines. The main ones are Bacteriology, or Medical Microbiology, with its later offshoots of Virology and Immunology; Histopathology, or Surgical Pathology, concerned with the microscopic study of tissues and cellular content of fluids, as well as post-mortem examinations; Haematology, the study of the blood and especially of its cellular components, including Blood Transfusion; and Clinical Chemistry, or Chemical Pathology, concerned with alterations in the chemical constitution of the blood and other fluids and tissues.

The provision of these diagnostic services at Bangour lagged far behind the establishment of clinical medicine and surgery. Before the formation of the NHS, the simpler diagnostic tests were performed in ward siderooms by junior doctors, or by 'laboratory assistants' who had no formal training but acquired their skills by example and experience, while for the more specialised investigations, Bangour remained heavily dependent on the old-established departments of Edinburgh University and Royal Infirmary.

In the early days a single laboratory, housed in what is now the Bacteriology Department, sufficed for the limited range of investigations then offered, mainly bacteriological. Gradual expansion in the scope of the work led to piecemeal acquisition of adjacent parts of the building, displacing the Pay Office, Accounts Department, Secretary and Treasurer to the Board of Management and Hospital Almoner. Until 1980 the telephone exchange persisted as a beleaguered enclave within the expanding laboratories but nevertheless provided a welcome source of cups of tea and gossip for laboratory personnel working outwith normal hours. Inroads were later made into the residential accommodation to the East of the main building, to house the burgeoning Haematology and Blood Transfusion Departments.

The laboratory was initially headed by Dr Isabella Purdie, who after training as a pharmacist had studied medicine and specialised in bacteriology. Mr James Tait was in technical charge and did much to raise the status of laboratory medicine at Bangour and elsewhere in the Lothians by lecturing and demonstrating at evening classes in Edinburgh until his premature death in 1974; he was succeeded by Mr Brian Lilley, who assumed technical charge of all the laboratories.

The Institute of Medical Laboratory Technology ran evening classes for trainees and held national examinations until the mid 1960s when responsibility was taken over by the Napier and Stevenson Colleges of Technology, students attending on a day-release basis and taking ONC and HNC examinations. Trainees at Bangour received practical experience in all laboratory disciplines before choosing one in which to specialise, but from the late 1970s the rapid expansion of laboratory medicine made this impracticable and new entrants were thereafter appointed to a single specialty. At about the same time it became fashionable for every artisan to adopt the name 'technician', and to protect their professional status Medical Laboratory Technicians changed their official title to Medical Laboratory Scientific Officers. Today's trainees study by day-release for a BSc degree in Life Sciences, a four-year course which embraces the theoretical aspects of all the medical laboratory disciplines.

General Practitioners made little use of the laboratory in its early days, but with the building of Health Centres in the main towns of West Lothian, staffed by young doctors who were experienced in using laboratory facilities, and the provision in the late 1960s of a daily van service, GPs found it increasingly easy to refer specimens to the laboratory, sometimes thereby obviating the need for an out patient appointment. The laboratory now serves twenty-one Health Centres, and the few specimens of the 1950s have grown to some 90,000 per annum.

In the early years specimens arrived from out patients in whatever container the patient thought suitable, jam jars and pill bottles being popular. One memorable specimen which provoked some hilarity contained a 24-hour collection of urine in a lemonade bottle bearing its original label emblazoned 'Mitchell's Sparkling Cola'. The name of the patient just happened to be Mitchell.

Until 1958 urgent out-of-hours specimens were dealt with by a member of the laboratory staff attending for an hour each evening and on Sunday mornings, to process any specimens left in the refrigerator. Outwith these times some investigations were still performed by the junior medical staff in ward siderooms. As the one hour evening visit gradually stretched to two or three and sometimes four hours, it became apparent that a round-the-clock service was required to give adequate emergency cover. Such a service was instituted in 1958, with one trained member of the laboratory staff on call each evening and at weekends, processing urgent specimens for bacteriological, haematological, blood transfusion and chemical analyses. Technical staff were still 'jacks-of-all-trades'. By the mid 1960s, demands were such that it was virtually impossible for one person to serve three disciplines adequately on an emergency basis, especially when a proportion of the calls were occasioned by the all too frequent head-on collisions on the 'Killer A8'. Thereafter Chemistry and Haematology and Blood Transfusion each provided an emergency service from their own staffs. A few of the older members in Bacteriology continued to take part in the Haematology/Blood Transfusion on-call rota until the early 1980s, when even they were overtaken by technological advances. At the time of writing the annual number of emergency calls outwith normal working hours has reached nearly 6,000, compared with around 300 in 1959.

As the laboratory workload continued to increase and gained in complexity the four disciplines became progressively less integrated, so that their development is better described separately.

BACTERIOLOGY

Much of the bacteriological work of the laboratory in the early years concerned the diagnosis of tuberculosis in its various forms. R9 housed the cases of tuberculous meningitis who were, in the main, children and young teenagers. They were subjected to the unpleasantness of having lumbar punctures performed each week for the purpose of obtaining cerebrospinal fluid, in which the causative organism could be found in the laboratory. Until the introduction of Streptomycin the outlook for these patients was bleak. The only antibiotics available for the treatment of non-tuberculous infections were the Sulphonamides, which had been in use for some years, and the more recently introduced Penicillin and Tetracycline. The potential effectiveness of these agents against a particular infection could be assessed by laboratory methods and the levels of antibiotic achieved in the patient's bloodstream monitored during treatment. During the 1960s and 1970s it seemed that a new antibiotic was being discovered every second month.

In the 1940s and 1950s the preparation of bacteriological culture media entailed the use of basic ingredients such as ox hearts from the abattoir and the slavish adherence to recipes which had changed little from the days of Louis Pasteur. Glassware was used exclusively throughout the laboratory and had to be decontaminated, washed and rinsed meticulously before re-use. Contaminated materials and utensils were immersed in 4-gallon enamel buckets of 10 per cent Lysol solution, which were then rendered completely germ-free by autoclaving. Before acquiring electrically heated autoclaves (quite simply a very much larger version of the present-day domestic pressure cooker), Bangour laboratory was the proud possessor of one heated by a Calor gas burner and another, even older, heated by means of an extremely temperamental Primus stove. However, a vast array of disposable plastic containers for laboratory use arrived on the scene during the 1960s and 1970s and this, in conjunction with the development of commercially prepared, dehydrated culture media, solved many difficulties but raised the new prob-lem of how to dispose of the disposables. By the mid 1950s the bacteriology section was examining milks from local dairies and Public Water supply samples. In 1956, the other sections of the laboratory having moved to their own accommodation, the bacteriology laboratory was extensively refur-bished, and included the installation of a central butane gas supply to replace the individual gas cylinders at each bunsen burner. The new system was tested for leaks by an engineer using a lighted wax taper—long before the days of the Health and Safety at Work Act.

When Dr Purdie retired in 1965, her reputation was such that she was made a founder Fellow of the Royal College of Pathologists. Dr Purdie was succeeded by Dr William McNaught from Peel Hospital, Galashiels, who became deeply involved in the setting up of the Regional Burns Unit at Bangour, the monitoring and control of infection being of prime importance in treating large burns. On his departure for Glasgow in 1972 he was replaced by Dr Raymond Wiseman, who continues to run the Bacteriology Lab for the West Lothian Hospitals and GPs.

HISTOPATHOLOGY

This was the last of the laboratory specialties to be established at Bangour. While the others existed, in however rudimentary a form, right from the beginning, histopathology continued to be the responsibility of the Edin-burgh University Pathology Department. Surgical pathology specimens were sent in batches to Edinburgh two or three times a week, resulting in delays which would not be acceptable nowadays and providing no opportunity for the close co-operation and consultation between surgeon and pathologist which is so essential to the proper interpretation of the findings. The temporary appointment of Dr Gavin Dunlop, a retired pathologist, in 1963 alleviated the latter problem but gave him little scope to establish the service since there was as yet no laboratory and all specimens still had to be sent to Edinburgh for processing.

Thereafter events moved with uncharacteristic swiftness. Dr Goldwyn Sclare, a Glaswegian languishing in Manchester, was appointed Consultant Pathologist in November 1964; Mr James Masson, just returned from Nigeria, was appointed Senior Technician, and a new laboratory extension was designed, built and in use by July 1965. Bangour clinicians now had a locally based service in surgical pathology and exfoliative cytology, as well as facilities for rapid frozen sections which provide an immediate diagnosis for a surgeon in the course of an operation. Although James Masson's tenure was short, he provided a firm foundation for the technical aspect of the service, which, from 1967, has remained in the charge of Mr Michael Coutts.

Provision of the new service unleashed a latent demand, so that the volume of work expanded rapidly, and the later development of fine-needle aspiration biopsy and immunohistochemistry added further to the number and range of investigations. In time the medical staff expanded to three, the technical staff to five and the secretarial staff to two. A succession of colourful assistants included Drs Louis Rosenthal, Margaret Pearson and Vincenzo Crucioli, and a second Consultant, Dr Ronald Davie from Dundee, was appointed in 1980. A spacious extension, doubling the size of the Department, was built in 1982. Dr Sclare retired in 1989, with Dr K Ramesar joining the staff to succeed him.

Post-mortem examinations, more commonly performed in the early days than now, took place in conditions which remained astonishingly primitive until a major reconstruction of the mortuary in 1978. Of the many stalwarts who served as mortuary attendants over the years, the most memorable was George Rea, to whom the task was an art as well as a science. By a mischance, of origin now unknown, the mortuary and post-mortem room were located in the first building to be encountered on entering the hospital, on the site of a previous piggery, instead of the usual discreet location beyond the vision of patients and visitors. The inevitable consequence was that the mortuary became a kind of unofficial hospital enquiry office. Many an innocent visitor was startled to find his enquiry answered by the mortuary attendant, whose attire proclaimed that he had been interrupted in the course of an autopsy.

HAEMATOLOGY AND BLOOD TRANSFUSION

In the 1950s the enumeration of blood cells, as an aid to the diagnosis of infections and anaemias, had to be performed manually using special glass pipettes and counting chambers examined microscopically. Early in the 1960s electronic cell-counting machines were introduced which enabled laboratories to process an ever-increasing workload, replacing time-consuming labour-intensive manual methods. The technological sophistication of present-day cell counters makes the original models seem archaic. The expertise of trained staff in the examination of stained smears of the blood and marrow for the diagnosis of anaemias, leukaemias and lymphomas is as yet resistant to automation.

In Blood Transfusion, methods existed for the identification of ABO blood groups, but it was not until the early 1950s that techniques were introduced for the determination of the Rhesus factor, which had only been discovered in 1948. It now seems with hindsight that previous to this discovery, the matching of patient to donor blood was rather a 'hit-or-miss' exercise. Advances in the knowledge and understanding of the complicated components of an individual's blood group have resulted in the matching of donor blood to patient now being undertaken with great confidence, and patients with certain blood disorders can now be transfused with specific factors extracted from donor blood.

Dr Margaret Cook was appointed Consultant Haematologist in 1976, replacing the part-time services of a haematologist from the Western General Hospital, Edinburgh. For the first time haematology was established as a discipline in its own right, differing from the other laboratory subjects in having combined laboratory and clinical responsibilities and providing, for both out-patient and in-patient, diagnosis and treatment of blood disorders.

CLINICAL CHEMISTRY

In the first ten to fifteen years the range of chemical investigations was limited, many depending on comparison of colours with standard colour discs which were to be read, according to the manufacturers' instructions, 'by a North light'. In the depths of winter certain investigations could not be performed after 4 p.m. However, in the early 1950s, an 'artificial daylight' lamp was produced with a blue bulb which solved that particular problem until the introduction of instruments with built-in illumination.

Dr L H Easson was appointed part-time Biochemist in 1953, dividing his time between the Royal Infirmary of Edinburgh, Bangour and Kirkcaldy, finally leaving Bangour in 1966 to remain as Biochemist at the new Victoria Hospital in Kirkcaldy. It is still remembered that on his first morning at Bangour no provision had been made for his arrival since no-one knew of his appointment, and Dr Purdie confessed to being considerably 'put out' at this lack of communication by the authorities. For three years his accommodation amounted to no more than a hastily-installed island bench in the middle of the bacteriology laboratory, a hostile environment in more ways than one.

By 1959 when Dr Ian Hendry joined Dr Easson as Senior Biochemist and there were two junior technical staff in post, all methods were still manual. Automation arrived at Bangour in 1962 with the purchase of an Autoanalyser, by which means the rate of chemical analyses could be increased from six to sixty per hour with the same number of staff. Automation and eventually computerisation have progressed steadily since then until the present day, when 600 tests per hour are possible. Dr Hendry was in sole charge of the department from 1966 to 1986 when Dr Derek McCullough was appointed Consultant Biochemist, under whose guidance the department now functions on two sites, at St John's and Bangour.

The opening of the first phase of the new hospital in 1989 entailed the departure to Livingston of the Haematology and Blood Transfusion departments, as well as a section of the Clinical Chemistry department, ending at a stroke both the close relationship of the four laboratories on a single site and the even more essential close relationship between the greater part of the laboratory staff and their clinical colleagues.

COMMUNITY SUPPORT

Bangour General and Village Hospitals have both benefited from the generosity of the people of West Lothian. The Staff in both hospitals have themselves raised funds for a wide variety of projects by means of prize draws, annual fetes, fashion shows, book sales, sponsored walks, bed pushes, parachute jumps, race nights and many other innovative methods. Two ambitious projects which required major fund raising appeals were the purchase of a custom built bus for the elderly disabled in 1978, costing £16,197, and the funding for two members of staff to attend a Cancer Conference in Melbourne, Australia in 1985.

Numerous donations have been received over the years from local companies, with the staff of the British Leyland Factory in Bathgate showing great generosity during the 1970s and both Levi Straus and Surgicos giving regular contributions during the 1980s. Many other organisations have given regular generous donations to the Bangour Hospitals, including the West Lothian Pigeon Show, the Local Round Table organisations and several of the local Orange Lodges.

During the war years, the Red Cross provided nursing services at Bangour General Hospital and in the late 1940s, initiated a trolley service selling confectionery and soft drinks to patients in all wards. This service was eventually taken over by the Women's Royal Voluntary Service (WRVS) and the Canteen by the bus stop at Bangour General Hospital was started in 1974 under the auspices of Mrs McKenzie, the District Organiser for West Lothian. Once the canteen was established a tea trolley was organised for the

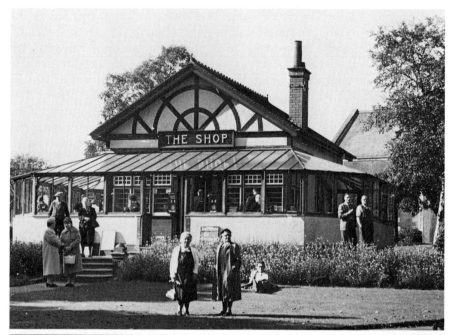

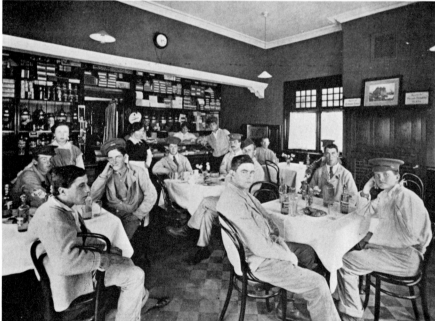

Fig. 69(a) and (b)   The Shop, Bangour Hospital, exterior (1950s) and interior (during the First World War).

out patient departments. This duty, over the years, has been carried out by a dedicated team of ladies in the various out patient clinics in P, Q, R and T blocks, ignoring rain, hail or snow and with or without all the wheels on the trolley working. In March 1966, Mrs Bunty Hamilton of Linlithgow became the West Lothian District Organiser to be followed by Mrs Betty Peat of Livingston, Mrs Sylvia Thom, and Mrs Moira Leitch was running the service when St John's Hospital at Howden was opened. The services provided by the WRVS are principally for the benefit of patients during their time in hospital but they are also utilised by hospital staff. Any profit made in the WRVS canteen or from the tea trolleys is given back to the hospitals in the District. Over the last twenty years, well over £20,000 has been donated to the Bangour Hospitals, as well as many gifts being presented, the first of which was bed curtains for the women's surgical ward in Q block, replacing portable screens.

In addition to organisations like the Women's Royal Voluntary Services and the Women's Rural Institute already mentioned in the history of the X-ray Department, there have been two very active League of Friends working in conjunction with the General and Village Hospitals. A similar League of Friends for St John's Hospital at Howden, Livingston was established in 1990 to ensure that the goodwill in the Community for the Bangour Hospitals is continued into the last decade of 1990s and the twenty-first century to support the development of St John's.

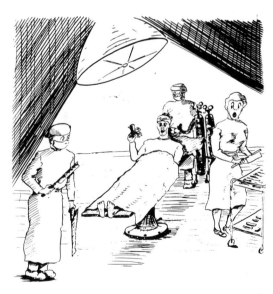

WOULD ANYONE CARE TO BUY A RAFFLE TICKET ?

Chapter Fourteen

The Bangour Annexe— The Final Years

Health care in West Lothian has come a long way since the days of the poor law institutions and isolation fever hospitals of the nineteenth century, the idealised Village community at the beginning of this century and the building of the war time annexe. Now St John's Hospital at Howden, Livingston is the latest step in that progression.

When the emergency medical services hospital was established at Bangour annexe in 1939, it was estimated that its temporary prefabricated buildings would last for ten, or at the most fifteen years. Following the war therefore, the people of West Lothian might reasonably have expected a new general hospital by 1955 or 1956 at the latest. Indeed, Dr J K Hunter, who was the first Director of the Scottish Hospital Advisory Service recounted that when he returned to Scotland in 1952 from the Colonial Service, the first task given to him by the Scottish Home and Health Department was to plan the new West Lothian General Hospital.

To begin with there were problems concerning the choice of site for the new hospital but the announcement by the Government in 1962 that Scotland's fifth and final official new town was to be at Livingston appears to have resolved this question. The choice of Livingston did not meet with the approval of all the Community in West Lothian. On 22 January 1965, the *Lothian Courier* carried a report headlined, '**Fight to keep Bangour**', in which Councillor J Kidd agreed that there was a need for a new hospital, but argued that it should be built at Bangour. He was backed by West Lothian County Convener, Peter Walker who stated: 'I read the report by the South East of Scotland Regional Health Board on the reasons for siting the new hospital at Livingston. Quite frankly, there is not a single argument in favour of such a move or any advantage that could not be put forward equally well for Bangour as a site. In fact Bangour has many more advantages'.

As the campaign to save Bangour gathered momentum, the *Courier* published an editorial on 7 July 1965, headed '**Room for Two**'. It suggested that while the new town of Livingston might eventually need a new hospital, there was still a need for one at Bangour to serve the rest of West Lothian.

Some of the heat was taken out of the argument early the following year when, on 11 February 1966, the *Courier* announced '**A reprieve for Bangour**'. The report stated: 'The arguments that have been raging the district since the Government announced its intention to replace Bangour with a new hospital in Livingston are likely to be abated because The Hospital Plan for Scotland stated that a new hospital for West Lothian had been deferred for at least five years'.

In the meantime, life went on as usual at Bangour until 18 December 1970 which was headlined in the *Courier* as a '**Red Letter Day as GP Unit Opens**'. This new Unit, which was the first of its kind in the South Eastern Region of Scotland (covering Lothians, Borders and Fife) was officially opened by the leading expert in Community Care, Professor John Brotherston who was later knighted for his services as Chief Medical Officer at the Scottish Home and Health Department. Professor Brotherston stressed that this new facility would further enhance the excellent work already being achieved as a result of the Livingston project of shared care between the hospital and the community described earlier in this book.

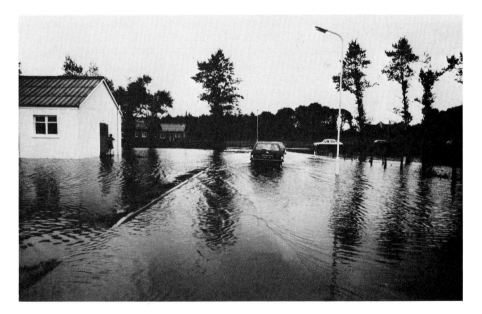

Fig. 70 In spite of frequent attempts to improve the drainage of the General Hospital, major flooding used to occur every couple of years. The level of water in the burn running through the centre of the Hospital was a very sensitive gauge to the amount of rainfall.

Dr Robert Milne, who is presently a General Practitioner working in Kirkliston, spent many years as a child living in a hospital house in Bangour. He remembers that

As a child in 1950, Bangour Hospital was my home and I can remember playing in the open spaces between the wards, enjoying the freedom that was denied to the patients, particularly those in R block, for that was where the victims of tuberculosis languished in bed for months on end. They were put out onto the open verandahs in the belief that fresh air might be therapeutic and I have vivid recollections of rows of beds in the open in all kinds of weather.

Coming to General Practice in West Lothian in 1976, I lost no time in getting myself a contract to use the GP unit, located in the very same block as those tuberculosis sufferers had occupied many years ago. By 1976, the verandahs had been glassed in and heated and the patients in these wards were in the direct care of their General Practitioners. Tuberculosis had been virtually eradicated by the development of Streptomycin and similar drugs.

John Brotherston was Chief Medical Officer at the Scottish Home and Health Department at the time of the development of Livingston new town, when the famous experiment with medical practice saw the introduction of Hospital Practitioners described earlier in this book. This was not the only initiative taken at that time because the General Practitioner Unit being opened in 1970 was specifically designed with the intention that interested General Practitioners would enhance the service to their patients by being able to bring them into hospital for investigations and treatment while the General Practitioner still retained overall clinical responsibility.

In 1990, it is important that we look back over these twenty years and try to decide whether the experiment has worked. The GP ward is still there and an enthusiastic but small number of doctors have established the reputation and proved the worth of this type of clinical care by using the Unit on a fairly active basis. There have been difficulties. The initial contract given to General Practitioners using the ward specified that doctors should only keep patients in the unit for a limited number of weeks, endeavouring to avoid the problem of 'blocked beds'. Unfortunately, the original spirit behind this recommendation was not always adhered to, and the management side of the hospital failed to enforce it, with the result that a gradual silting up of the GP Unit facilities took place, beds becoming blocked with inappropriately admitted patients. The effect of this was to reduce the availability of facilities for genuine users and consequently there was a loss of enthusiasm among some of the General Practitioners.

Nevertheless, the spirit of the enterprise lives on and with the coming of the new hospital in Livingston, a commitment has been made by the hospital management that there will be a General Practitioner Unit in Phase 2 of St John's Hospital at Howden. Accordingly, Professor Sir John Brotherston's initiative of 1970 has been sustained and experience has shown that there is a place in modern medical practice for this kind of service where General Practitioners can extend the care they provide for appropriate patients by admitting them to a hospital bed with a view to making use of the hospital's resources.

Even with new facilities such as the General Practitioner ward and a constant round of upgrading, Bangour was beginning to show its age by the late 1970s. Livingston was steadily becoming more established in West Lothian as an integral part of the Community and the building of its excellent road network readily linked the new town with other areas in the county. All these factors meant that there was much less opposition than had occurred a decade earlier, when it was announced in 1974, that approval had been given in principal to build a new 690 bed hospital at Howden, Livingston. Initially it was proposed to build the replacement for Bangour General Hospital in one phase at a cost of 11.8 million pounds. Almost at the same time, however, the Operational Research Unit of the Department of Health issued a report indicating that all hospitals on new sites should be built in phases as small as possible, allowing for medical, operating and design considerations, as this would prevent over provision of services in the early stages and avoid excess of expenditure.

This proposal to phase the replacement for Bangour General Hospital was strongly supported by the Project Team made up of representatives from the Building Division of the Common Services Agency of the Scottish Home and Health Department, whose officers included Architects, Engineers, Surveyors, Medical and Nursing advisers. The Lothian Health Board's officers on the project team were Dr W A Simpson, Community Medicine Specialist, Miss G M Daniels, District Nursing Officer and Mr K Rankine, Assistant Secretary of the Capital Services Division.

With the famous Livingston Health Services project in mind, the Project Team agreed that a large, full scale Health Centre would be an integral part of the site of the major District General Hospital they were planning. To begin with, three phases were planned: the first and second phases were designed to replace the General Hospital, allowing an expansion in general medical service. The proposed third phase was to enable Bangour Village Hospital to be closed, but the management of psychiatric illness and the increasing emphasis on community based services soon threw doubt on whether a third phase would ever be required.

As always Bangour was leading the way in the treatment of patients with mental disorders and its provisions for such patients were increased in 1976 with the opening of Bangour Village Hospital's own modern factory workshop, costing £154,000. In this sheltered workshop, both in and out patients were encouraged to regain their skills with the eventual aim of enabling them to return to their normal working situation. The workshop was officially opened by Mr Tam Dalyell, MP, who praised the concept of allowing patients to undertake contracts for commercially viable products, ranging from wooden toys to garden sheds.

Bangour again hit the national headlines in 1978 when staff secretly entered Charge Nurse Elizabeth Brown in the *Scottish Daily Express* Nurse of the Year competition. In the televised final, Elizabeth, from Knightsridge in Livingston, walked off with the title. Elizabeth said, 'I nearly fainted when I found out I had been entered for the competition. Now, however, I am very happy because winning is such a wonderful boost for Bangour.'

With such tremendous loyalty to the hospital, it was natural that there was a touch of sadness as well as pride when it was announced in 1981 that work on the new hospital was, at last, actually going to start on the site at Howden in Livingston. In June 1981 what was described as 'advance work' began. The first building to go up was a 5.2 million pound fully automated laundry to replace the old Edwardian one at the Village Hospital. At the same time a massive modern coal fired boiler house was built. Coal was the preferred type of fuel, because of the close links in West Lothian with the mining industry. Regretably these links died with the closure of Polkemmet Colliery in 1988. The other building to be started at that time was the new Howden Health Centre, confirming that it was intended to play an integral part in the planning of the new hospital. This Health Centre remains a lasting confirmation of the success of the Livingston Health Service project.

In January 1983, building started on Phase 1 of the hospital. The Main Contractors being Melville, Dundas and Whitson and the Architects Boswell, Mitchell and Johnstone. The years 1985 and 1986 saw a period of great turmoil with regard to the planning of Phase 1 and Phase 2 of the hospital. West Lothian Unit Management were anxious to formally establish a Phase 1 Commissioning Team as soon as possible but decisions were delayed until the Scottish Home and Health Department obtained assurances from the Lothian Health Board with regard to the revenue consequences of building and opening the massive Phase 1 hospital building project. One possibility that arose during these deliberations was the proposal that only part of the development would take place, thus minimising both capital and revenue costs. The main controversy that arose at this time concerned the development of a Paediatric Unit in the new hospital. Mr John McKay, MP, Conservative Minister of Health at the Scottish Office confirmed to the House of Commons that such a Unit would open, following a parliamentary question by Robin Cook, MP—the Labour Member of Parliament for Livingston. It was immediately recognised, although not widely accepted by all parties across the Lothian Health Board, that such a development would require radical realignment of paediatric services throughout the Lothian

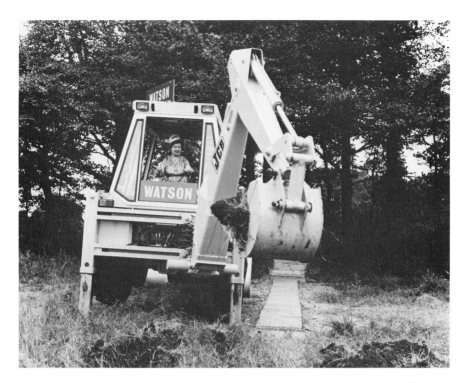

Fig. 71 Dr Rina Nealon, Chairman of the Lothian Health Board, cut the first sod at the site in Howden, Livingston, where the new hospital replacing Bangour General was to be built.

The South East of Scotland Regional Hospital Board first announced plans for the new hospital in 1965, but it was 1974 before 'approval in principle' was given to go ahead with the plans, 1981 when building started and 28 October 1989 when the first patient entered Phase 1 of St John's Hospital at Howden, Livingston.

region, to the great benefit of the children of West Lothian who would no longer have to travel to Edinburgh for paediatric care.

At last, in the autumn of 1986, formal authority was given by the Lothian Health Board to commence the commissioning process for Phase 1 of the new hospital. Any commissioning process is a major undertaking and its timing was crucial if the bricks and mortar of the building were to be translated into a functioning hospital able to provide high standards of clinical care to the patients of West Lothian. The commissioning process involved major decisions about which services would move to Phase 1 of St John's Hospital and apparently minor decisions as to how many wash hand basins would be available in the new hospital. The first permanent members of staff on the Commissioning Team were appointed in December 1986—the

Commissioning Officer was Miss Alison Baxter and the Commissioning Nurse Miss Rosemary Torrance. These two members of staff, working with Miss Jan Robinson for Nursing, Mr Donald Macleod, representing the Medical Staff and Mr Paul Lynch from the Hospital Management, were the driving force behind the commissioning process, ensuring that the building schedule and plans for patients moving into the hospital in late 1989 were achieved.

One area in which the Commissioning team faced great controversy was in choosing a name for the new hospital. After considerable debate within the hospital and community in West Lothian, the name of St John's Hospital at Howden, Livingston was recommended by the Lothian Health Board to the Scottish Home and Health Department. This choice of name reflects the very early provision of health care within West Lothian and beyond, by the order of the Knights of St John of Jerusalem. This historic order, which reaches back to the twelfth century, has its Scottish headquarters and priory at Torphichen in West Lothian. In addition, the new hospital has been built in close proximity to land previously leased to the Order at Knightsridge.

This commissioning process was successfully accomplished and Phase 1 of St John's Hospital at Howden was opened to receive its first patients on 30 October 1989. The first admissions were Marie Hamilton of East Calder and Jacky Henderson of Bathgate, both of whom were presented with a small momento of the occasion by Mr Paul Taylor, General Manager of the West Lothian Unit.

Phase 1 of the new hospital was occupied by the following specialties: General Surgery, Orthopaedics, Ear, Nose and Throat surgery, Obstetrics and Gynaecology, Special Care Baby Unit, General Medicine, Geriatric Assessment Unit, Accident and Emergency Department and the new Paediatric or Children and Young Persons ward. In addition to these clinical services the main X-ray Department and Haematology Laboratories were transferred to St John's. The Regional Plastic Surgery and Burns Unit with the Oral Surgery Department, Physiotherapy, the General Practitioner ward and the Geriatric services were all left at Bangour Hospital with the Pathology, Bacteriology and Biochemistry Laboratories. These services will move to Phase 2 of the new hospital which was officially 'topped out' on 12 January 1990. The ceremony was organised by John Laing and Company, the Main Contractors for Phase 2 and the 'topping out' was carried out by Mr Bruce Weatherstone, Chairman of the Lothian Health Board. It is anticipated that Phase 2 of the hospital will be fully commissioned and ready for patients in the spring of 1992. In addition to the services already identified, Phase 2 will also accommodate 100 acute Psychiatric and Psychogeriatric assessment beds and a Unit for the Young Chronic Sick in conjunction with rehabilitation medicine.

The official opening of St John's Hospital at Howden, which at one stage

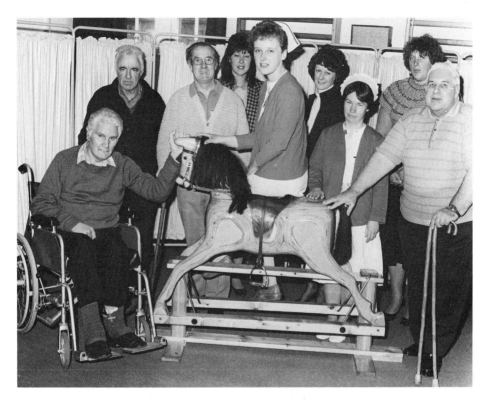

Fig. 72   Patients at Winchburgh Day Hospital presented this magnificent wooden rocking horse to the large numbers of children attending the Ear Nose and Throat Department in Bangour. The patients made the horse from layered plywood before it was carved and decorated. The rocking horse has found a permanent home in the Children's Ward in St John's Hospital at Howden.

The photograph shows Danny McFarlane and a group of patients presenting the horse to Staff Nurse Robertson, Sister Dowditch and Catherine McMillan from the ENT Ward. In the background Alison Baxter, on the left, and Rosemary Torrance were present as the key members of the commissioning team equipping the new hospital.

was the largest hospital building project in Europe, was undertaken by Her Majesty The Queen, accompanied by His Royal Highness, Prince Philip, on Thursday, 12 July 1990. This brought to a successful conclusion a sequence of planning and investment that started in the mid 1950s and now stands as a memorial to the much loved and respected Bangour Annexe or General Hospital and the many individuals who have served Bangour while at the same time ensuring the development of St John's.

Hospital administration in West Lothian, starting with the formation of the National Health Service in 1948, was under the auspices of a Board of

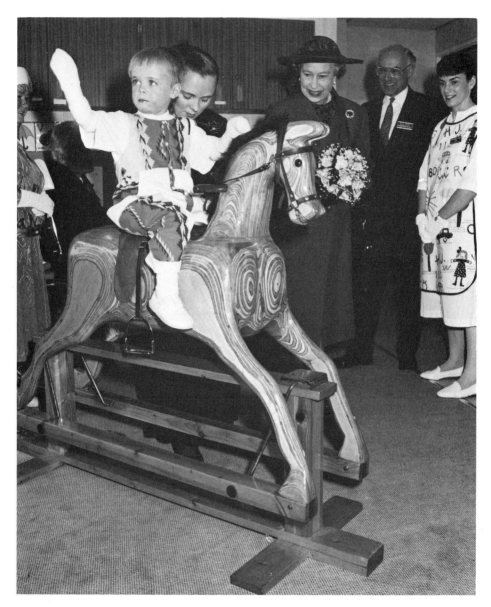

Fig. 73 Opening Day, St John's. Her Majesty the Queen officially opened St John's Hospital at Howden, Livingston on 12 July 1990. During the Queen's visit to the new Children's Ward she was able to see the hand-made rocking horse being used by Sean Glen. The Ward Sister, Susan Milne, and Consultant Paediatrician Dr Gordon Stark, accompanied the Queen on her tour of the ward. The Duke of Edinburgh was also present at the opening ceremony, visiting many departments in the Hospital.

Management. It was initially chaired by Lieutenant Colonel J Kidd, a Solicitor and Partner in the Company of Peterkin and Kidd, WS, Solicitors of Linlithgow. The Hospital Board of Management was responsible to the South East of Scotland Regional Hospital Board which co-ordinated Health Care Services in Fife, Lothian and Borders on the basis of tripartite structure separating hospitals, General Practice and Community Medical Services.

This structure was dismantled in one of the many re-organisations of Scottish Health Service administration that has taken place in the fifty years since Bangour General Hospital was established. In 1974, the South East of Scotland Regional Hospital Board was sub-divided into three separate Health Boards, for Fife, the Borders and the Lothians. The West Lothian District was established as part of the Lothian Health Board and, with Mr Alex Maltman as District Administrator was given the task of unifying the previous tripartite system for Hospital, General Practice and Community Medical Services. The concept of the West Lothian District providing integrated medical services was extremely attractive as the district boundary coincided with the boundaries of West Lothian and therefore a natural geographic entity was established.

The West Lothian district survived the immense re-organisation of Health Service administration which took place in 1984 which was involved in establishing General Management with a view to giving a more purposeful leadership to the integrated health services. West Lothian Unit, as it is now known, remained intact and when Mr Alex Maltman retired as District Administrator, he was replaced by Mr Paul Taylor as the West Lothian Unit General Manager. Throughout these challenging and changing times of Health Service administration, provision of innovative and integrated medical services in the Bangour Hospitals has been facilitated by a wide and varied group of administrators and their support staff who have recognised the unique geographical entity of West Lothian and have served the Community by promoting the development of very high standards of medical care.

Appendix

REQUIEM FOR A WARD

At 8 a.m. the morning ward round proceeded without incident. There were fewer patients than usual but most were ill. There was, however, a discernible holiday atmosphere—like Christmas without decorations.

At 4 p.m. the ward was dead, empty for the first time in half a century. It will never again be opened for patients. The fabric will rot through neglect before being pulled down and the site resold or reclaimed for some as yet undecided purpose. No trace will remain of what was once one of the busiest and most innovative general surgical wards in Scotland, which had shared with other outwardly more prestigious units the distinction of being depicted on the cover of the *British Journal of Surgery*. Only memories will remain—those of tens of thousands of patients who passed through it and those of the relatively few surgeons privileged to work there.

This was an old fashioned unpretentious Florence Nightingale ward where the bed state and the degree of nursing and medical activity could be assessed at a glance through the scarred opaque plastic swing doors opening into it. It was really only a hut, like hundreds of others put up in 1939 to cope with the casualties expected from the forthcoming conflict and designed to last for five years. The hut leaked when it rained, was drafty and noisy when the wind blew, and sweltered in the sun. That it was, nevertheless, a happy and fulfilling place in which to practise surgery was a tribute to the nurses and paramedical staff who combined to produce an attitude of caring, coping, and getting the job done. The open Nightingale ward stimulated the patients to support and encourage each other through personal worries and clinical crises. This collective pooling of emotional strength may have been largely responsible for their almost unbelievable bravery in the face of the frightening, humiliating, and painful circumstances which can be the lot of the patient admitted for surgery.

Now the 25 beds were empty, mattresses stripped and clustered at the end of the ward. Rubbish bags of various hues lay around in untidy profusion. Desks had been rifled, wall fixtures removed, and cupboards emptied. The eye was drawn to the tattiness of the décor—peeling paint, cracked windows, and buckled linoleum. The ward had been gutted and was now nothing more than a cold, abandoned, dirty hut. Standing there in the dead silence of what had been my first consultant charge, I was surprised by a sense of desolation.

That day we had completed the move to our brave new hospital, a much awaited event and heralded as a great achievement for the NHS in Scotland. One of our patients marked the occasion by bleeding again from his duodenal ulcer during the four and a half km transfer journey.

Three surgical wards have been combined into one 72 bedded flat of modern state of the art configuration with a central high dependency and intensive care unit, flanked by two wings containing six bedded bays and single rooms. The décor is wonderful—Regency striped wallpaper, tasteful curtains and screens, beautiful hardwood fittings, and a light blue carpet. At least the carpet *was* nice. Unfortunately, despite assurances to the contrary, stains do not come out. Our problems with surgical spillages are nothing compared with those of the obstetric and paediatric wards. Apparently, carpets need less cleaning than linoleum and fewer domestic staff are required; hence we have stained carpets and great efficiency.

The loss of the open plan ward is difficult to adjust to. Patients have to be moved about the unit regularly producing confusion for them, their relatives, and their medical attendants. A great deal of ward round time is now spent in tracking down the patients. For an elective colonic resection the patient will be admitted to a single room with a toilet for bowel preparation before operation, will return from the theatre to the high dependency or intensive care unit before, if all goes well, moving on to convalesce in one of the six bedded bays out in the wings. He or she may consequently have passed through the hands of up to three different nursing charges. Continuity of nursing care seems no longer possible.

Deciding where to put patients in this surgical maze is a problem. The young patient with early breast cancer incarcerated in a bay with two jaundiced old ladies with inoperable malignancies seems inappropriate. We would not wish such a patient to consider herself particularly ill nor would we want to confront her with the possible outcome of her disease. In the previous ward she could have found other women of her own age and perhaps similar problems and would have gained support and comfort, not immediately evident in the new system. Should she venture out of her area looking for company, she will probably wander into the men's bay. Not all our patients are ready for mixed wards. Most men find catheters embarrassing enough without having to expose them and themselves to women of all ages.

Counselling patients in six bedded bays is impossible. Everyone in the room can listen in. By contrast, it was perfectly possible to have a private conversation in the midst of the bustle of the old Nightingale ward. Putting such patients in single rooms does not necessarily solve the problem and can make the lonely, introspective patient feel isolated and brood excessively. The open ward offered the patient the chance to withdraw or to interact with others to a variable degree on a day to day basis.

We are coming to terms with these deficiencies in the design of our new ward and are cranking up our surgical unit to an acceptable level of efficiency. In time, we may come to hold this place in the same regard as we did its predecessor. Nevertheless, our hospital move has proved stressful for many of its staff who feel a lingering sense of anticlimax. Those who still work in ancient hospitals in old fashioned Florence Nightingale wards may be better off than they think.

J B RAINEY

(BMJ, Vol. 300, 9 May 1990)

Index